Low flow anaesthesia

To my wife Hilde
and my children Antje and Jan

Low flow anaesthesia

The theory and practice of low flow, minimal flow and closed system anaesthesia

Jan A. Baum   Priv Doz Dr med
Department of Anaesthesia and Intensive Medicine, Krankenhaus St Elisabeth-Stift, Damme, Germany

English text revised by

Geoffrey Nunn BA(Hons) MB BS FRCA
Consultant Anaesthetist, Pinderfields Hospital, Wakefield, UK

With a Foreword by **Peter Lawin** Prof Dr med Dr hc, FCCM
em. Chairman, Klinik und Poliklinik für Anaesthesiologie und operative Intensivmedizin, University of Münster, Germany

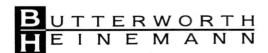

Butterworth-Heinemann
Linacre House, Jordan Hill, Oxford OX2 8DP
A division of Reed Educational & Professional Publishing Ltd

 A member of the Reed Elsevier plc group

OXFORD LONDON BOSTON
NEW DELHI SINGAPORE SIDNEY
TOKYO TORONTO WELLINGTON

Original German version 1988, 1992
Revised English version 1996

British Library Cataloguing in Publication Data
A catalogue record for this book
is available from the British Library

ISBN 0 7506 2127 3

Typeset by P&R Typesetters Ltd, Salisbury, Wiltshire.
Printed and bound by Hartnolls Ltd, Bodmin, Cornwall

Contents

Foreword

The dominant question is no longer whether to use a closed circuit but how to use it safely.
(H. J. Lowe and E. A. Ernst, 1981)

Methods of anaesthesia with reduced fresh gas flows, up to the technique of 'quantitative anaesthesia' with a completely closed rebreathing system, have gained more and more interest in recent years. The present high standard of medical equipment, the potential for continuous and comprehensive analysis of anaesthetic gas composition, mandatory safety standards for anaesthetic equipment, and increased knowledge of the pharmacokinetics and pharmacodynamics of the inhalational anaesthetics justify the revival of these methods. This calls for a reappraisal of anaesthetic practice since, with a reduction of the fresh gas flow, the gas composition within the breathing system is increasingly determined by the technical and constructional characteristics of the particular breathing system, by the pharmacokinetic properties of the volatile anaesthetics and the individual patient's oxygen consumption, rather than by the composition of the fresh gas itself. Thus, the practical performance of anaesthesia with reduced fresh gas flow requires intense study of technical details, regularities of oxygen and inhalation anaesthetic uptake, and the fundamentals of organ transfer and elimination of anaesthetic gases.

This book, presented by J. Baum, is one of the few monographs on anaesthetic methods with reduced fresh gas flow providing a comprehensive overview of the subject. Following discussion of theoretical fundamentals, the author refers in detail to problems and questions arising in the practical performance of these methods. The information on technical details and legal considerations refers to up-to-date equipment standards and relevant regulations.

Discussion on technical practicality, the potential perspectives of comprehensive non-invasive patient monitoring, and the clinical significance of quantitative anaesthesia is still continuing. However, there can be no doubt that, apart from all known advantages, the concern about anaesthesia with low fresh gas flow intensifies the need for the understanding of equipment function and the pharmacology of inhalational anaesthesia. This is not only an advantage with respect to mastering this anaesthetic method, but is very much also to the benefit of patient safety. Increasing utilization of rebreathing and the reduction of unused excess anaesthetic gas by electronic control of both volume and gas composition in the breathing system will doubtless become the technical concept of future generations of anaesthetic machines. This book is recommended because of its exceptionally clear didactic concept and its straightforwardly structured, but nevertheless extensive presentation of this subject. It deserves to be widely read: the interesting and useful methods of anaesthesia with low fresh gas flow will increasingly be applied in daily hospital routine.

Peter Lawin

Preface to the English edition

As the fundamental books on low flow anaesthetic techniques (H. J. Lowe and E. A. Ernst's *The Quantitative Practice of Anesthesia* and J. A. Aldrete, H. J. Lowe and R. W. Virtue's *Low Flow and Closed System Anesthesia*) are already more than ten years old, it seems justified to submit a new English textbook, comprehensively describing the different aspects of anaesthesia with reduced fresh gas flow from a current point of view. Due to more stringent regulations on occupational safety and health, an increasing environmental awareness, the development of highly advanced anaesthetic machines and the demand for economical use of anaesthetic gases, there is an increasing interest in this subject. More and more anaesthetists are becoming aware of the absurd anachronism that the majority of anaesthetic machines feature technically advanced rebreathing systems and monitoring devices but are mostly used with fresh gas flows which virtually exclude any rebreathing. Actually, a widespread acceptance of low flow anaesthetic techniques is not hindered by insufficient technical equipment but much more by lack of experience and a reluctance to learn new techniques.

The reason for reservations towards anaesthetic techniques with low fresh gas flow is based on the fact that the majority of anaesthetists are unfamiliar with these methods, and there is great uncertainty with respect to dosage of anaesthetic gases and the suitability of available anaesthetic machines for these methods. In addition, there are still concerns about process-inherent hazards such as accidental hypoxia and overdose of volatile anaesthetics.

It is the objective of this book, which deals with the different variants of anaesthesia with reduced fresh gas flow with regard to practicability and assurance of patient safety, to clarify the specific problems of these anaesthetic techniques and available equipment. At the same time, it should overcome unjustified reservations by giving practical advice on the performance of these methods.

I wish to thank my esteemed clinical and academic teacher, Prof. Dr med Dr h.c. Peter Lawin, FCCM, em. Chairman and Director of the Klinik und Poliklinik für Anaesthesiologie und operative Intensivmedizin at the University of Münster for his continuous and benevolent support of my clinical and scientific work. The author's own investigations on minimal flow anaesthesia, which include a vast number of individual measurements, could not have been accomplished without the assistance of my colleagues, Chief Physician Dr med G. Sachs and the Senior Anaesthetists Dr med Ch. von den Driesch and Dr med G. Stanke. I feel greatly obliged for their committed assistance. This also goes for the anaesthetic nursing staff of the author's department, K. Luzak, U. Kramer, Th. Krausse and W. Weitzmann, who took a great interest in the technical details of anaesthetic machines, this being an indispensable requirement for safe performance of this anaesthetic technique. I owe special gratitude to the chief anaesthetic nurse, R. Prior, who made great contributions in preparing the chapter on equipment maintenance. Furthermore, I wish to thank all those who have accompanied my work with essential discussions and benevolent criticism, providing valuable advice on many question of detail. This especially applies to all discussions concerning detail problems with Dr med L. Atzmüller, Linz, and with Dr M. Graw and Dr C. F. Wallroth, Lübeck. In preparing the illustrations and flow diagrams of anaesthetic machines, I received generous support from the different manufacturers. The first draft of the English translation of the book's German edition was made by Mrs H. Eicke, Lübeck. Whenever there was urgent need for literature and texts of other authors, I could always rely on instant help from Mrs H. Blohm, Mrs A. Averbeck, Mrs C. Bromby and Mrs A. Tewes from Prof. Lawin's office. Last but not least I have to thank Dr Geoffrey Nunn for his excellent revision of the English text. Dr Nunn not only succeeded in transforming the rough original text into smooth English but also made several amendments and corrections essentially improving its content.

Jan Baum

Introduction

The rapid advance in the development of the technology of anaesthetic machines, more stringent regulations on occupational safety, growing awareness in matters of environmental protection, and the demand for economical use of anaesthetic gases worldwide were the reasons for producing an English version of the book *Praxis der Minimal Flow Anaesthesie*, which was first published in 1988, with a revised second edition in 1992.

The subject is approached with a detailed classification of breathing systems, giving consideration to both technical and functional criteria. This is followed by a discussion on the historical development of different breathing systems and their different methods of use. Pharmacokinetics of anaesthetic gases, the uptake of oxygen during the course of anaesthesia and the different anaesthetic methods with low fresh gas flows are dealt with in detail. The rules and guidelines according to which inhalation anaesthesia has to be controlled at differing fresh gas flows will be demonstrated with the aid of computer simulations and clinical measurements. Five pharmacokinetic simulation programs will be described in detail, since this will aid the understanding of particularities in low flow anaesthesia, thus facilitating the learning process on the characteristics of this anaesthetic technique. In discussing the advantages of rebreathing, not only is the reduction in anaesthetic gas consumption and costs dealt with, but also the improvement of anaesthetic gas climate. With growing environmental awareness and stiffer regulations on occupational safety and health, the reduction in anaesthetic gas emissions becomes an ever important aspect.

Two extensive chapters are dedicated to technical requirements and performance of low flow anaesthesia, including the necessary monitoring. A number of anaesthetic machines and monitoring systems are described in detail and evaluated with respect to technical concepts and practical clinical use. Highly advanced equipment, by means of which quantitative closed system anaesthesia can be carried out, will also be presented. Evaluation of low flow anaesthesia in relation to patient safety is of great clinical relevance. A special section is devoted not only to method-inherent risks but also to method-inherent safety features.

The chapter on the practice of minimal flow anaesthesia comprehensively explains the practical performance of this anaesthetic method, by means of which the fresh gas flow can be reduced to the greatest possible extent when using semi-closed rebreathing systems. Practical advice is given with respect to maintenance and care of anaesthetic machines. Recommendations on appropriate adjustment of fresh gas composition, dosage of volatile anaesthetics, induction, emergence and maintenance of anaesthesia, are made in line with experience gained during the performance of minimal flow anaesthesia in clinical practice.

Finally, the book presents an outlook on future developments. Progress seems to point towards the appropriate utilization of rebreathing systems by reduction of the fresh gas flow. Anaesthetists will have to keep pace with this trend and include inhalational anaesthesia with low fresh gas flow in their clinical repertoire and practical routine.

Symbols and abbreviations

AD_{95}	Anaesthetic concentration at which 95% of all patients tolerate skin incision without any motoric reaction
aeD_{CO_2}	Arterial-end expiratory carbon dioxide partial pressure difference
APV	Alternating pressure ventilation
BET	Bouls–Elimination–Transfer (pharmacokinetic scheme)
BW (kg)	Body weight in kg
C_A	Alveolar concentration
C_a	Arterial concentration
C_{CO}	Carbon monoxide concentration
C_i	Inspired concentration
DGAI	German Society for Anaesthesiology and Intensive Care Medicine
ECG	Electrocardiogram
E:I	Expiratory–inspiratory ratio
F_A	Alveolar fraction
F_D	Delivered fraction
F_E	Expired fraction
FGF	Fresh gas flow (see also $\dot{V}_f$)
FGU	Fresh gas utilisation
F_I	Inspired fraction
FiO_2	Fraction inspired oxygen
FiN_2O	Fraction inspired nitrous oxide
IPPV	Intermittent positive pressure ventilation
ISO	International Standards Organisation
ITN	Anasthesia with endotracheal intubation
I_{tox}	Toxicity index
K_D	Cumulative dose
kg	Kilogram
$\lambda_{B/G}$	Blood gas partition coefficient
$\lambda_{T/B}$	Tissue blood partition coefficient
MAC	Minimum alveolar concentration
MAK	Maximum workplace concentration
min	Minutes
MV	Minute volume
ORC	Oxygen ratio controller
p	Pressure
$Paco_2$	Arterial carbon dioxide partial pressure

P_D	Prime dose
$PeCO_2$	End expiratory carbon dioxide partial pressure
PEEP	Positive end expiratory pressure
$\dot{Q}$	Cardiac output
$\dot{Q}_{eff}$	Efficiency quotient
$\dot{Q}_T$	Tissue (organ) blood flow
r	Respiratory (ventilation) rate
SIMV	Synchronized intermittent mandatory ventilation
t	Time
T	Time constant
T_V	Tidal volume
U_D	Unit dose
$\dot{V}CO_2$	Carbon dioxide production
VA	Volatile anaesthetic
V_A	Alveolar volume
$\dot{V}_A$	Alveolar minute volume
$\dot{V}_{AN}$	Anaesthetic uptake
VE	Ventilation
$\dot{V}_f$	Fresh gas flow
$\dot{V}_{if}$	Fresh gas flow during inspired phase
$\dot{V}_{fN_2O}$	Nitrous oxide flow
VIC	Vaporization inside the circle
$\dot{V}_{N_2O}$	Nitrous oxide uptake
VOC	Vaporizer outside uptake
$\dot{V}_{O_2}$	Oxygen uptake (oxygen consumption)
$\dot{V}_{fO_2}$	Oxygen flow
V_L	Volume of the patient's lung
V_S	Volume of the system (breathing system, gas reservoir, ventilator)
V_T	Tissue (organ) volume
$\dot{V}_U$	Uptake
ZEEP	Zero end expiratory pressure

Breathing systems – technical concepts and function

Breathing systems are the technical elements of anaesthetic machines by means of which anaesthetic gas is administered to the patient. This makes them the technical link between the patient and the apparatus which provides the fresh gas. Being also influenced by ventilation parameters, constructive principles, and the specific apparatus design, the composition of the anaesthetic gas depends mainly upon the breathing system's technical design and the fresh gas flow.

1.1 Classification of breathing systems according to underlying technical concepts

Based on the technical concept, and in accordance with the nomenclature recommended by E. A. Ernst[1] and the International Standards Organisation (ISO)[2], breathing systems can be divided into three main groups (Figure 1.1).

1.1.1 Rebreathing systems

Rebreathing systems are characterized by the rerouting of the expired gas, admixed with fresh gas, back to the patient during the following inspiratory phase. In this process it is essential that uncontrolled carbon dioxide enrichment is prevented. This means that devices which eliminate carbon dioxide from the expired gas must be made an indispensable and integral part of such systems.

In satisfying this requirement, the to-and-fro and the circle absorption systems, which are designed as rebreathing systems, are equipped with carbon dioxide absorbers.

The most commonly used rebreathing system is the circle absorption system, because to-and-fro absorption systems are not very convenient and are unreliable with respect to carbon dioxide elimination, since the dead space of the system increases during use in parallel with the exhaustion of the soda lime.

The classification and terminology concerning breathing systems as given by Davey *et al.*[10] are incompatible with common usage and ISO terminology[2]. Great efforts should be made to standardize the terminology concerning breathing systems so as to facilitate international scientific exchange.

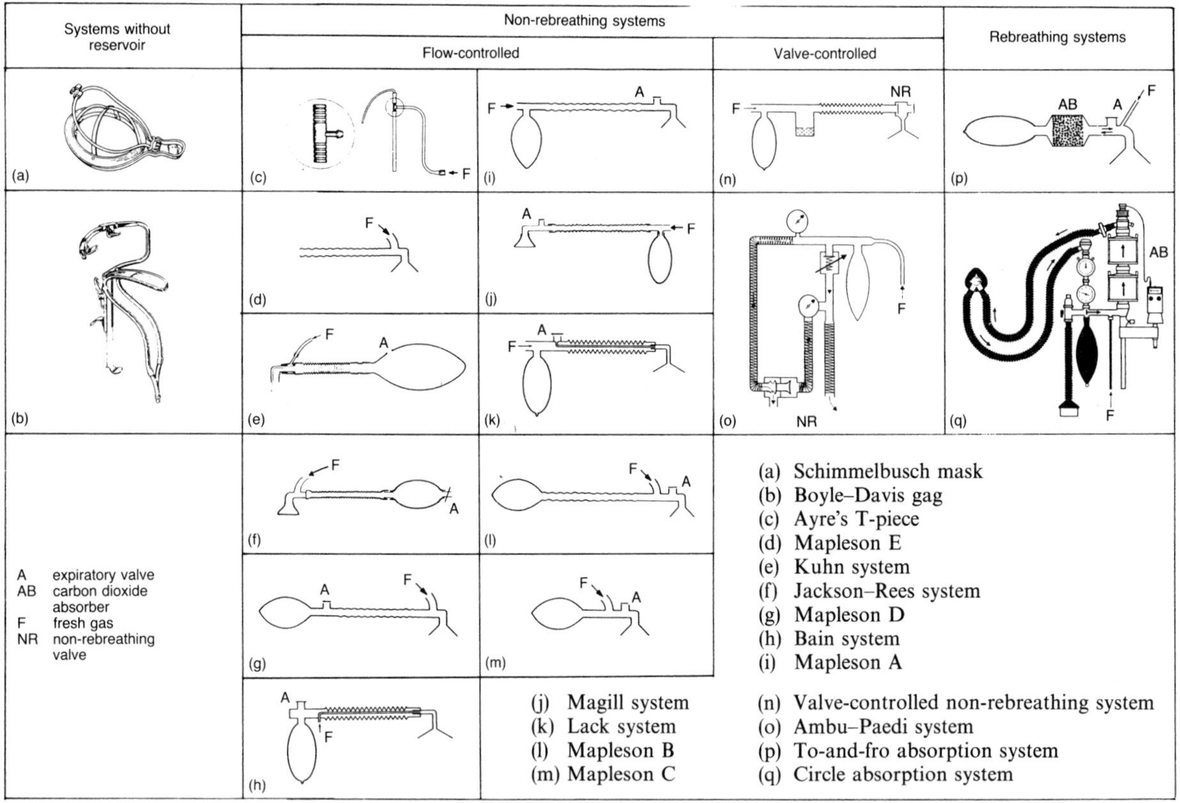
Systems without reservoir
Non-rebreathing systems
Flow-controlled
Valve-controlled
Rebreathing systems
(a)
(b)
(c)
(d)
(e)
(f)
(g)
(h)
(i)
(j)
(k)
(l)
(m)
(n)
(o)
(p)
(q)
A
F
NR
AB
A expiratory valve
AB carbon dioxide absorber
F fresh gas
NR non-rebreathing valve
(a) Schimmelbusch mask
(b) Boyle–Davis gag
(c) Ayre's T-piece
(d) Mapleson E
(e) Kuhn system
(f) Jackson–Rees system
(g) Mapleson D
(h) Bain system
(i) Mapleson A
(j) Magill system
(k) Lack system
(l) Mapleson B
(m) Mapleson C
(n) Valve-controlled non-rebreathing system
(o) Ambu–Paedi system
(p) To-and-fro absorption system
(q) Circle absorption system

Figure 1.1 (a–q) Synoptic presentation of breathing systems, classified according to their basic technical concept (From References 3–9)

1.1.2 Non-rebreathing systems

Technically, non-rebreathing systems are designed such that the entire expired gas, or at least the carbon dioxide containing alveolar ventilation volume, is removed from the system and replenished by fresh gas. There are two technical concepts which satisfy this requirement.

With valve-controlled non-rebreathing systems (Figure 1.2a), the entire expired gas is discharged into the atmosphere via a non-rebreathing valve arranged close to the mask or tube connector. The patient inhales pure fresh gas from the inspiratory limb of the system. Rebreathing is impossible because of this control principle.

With flow-controlled non-rebreathing systems, the expired gas is displaced from the system by a sufficiently high fresh gas flow. This method is made possible because the inspiratory limb of these systems is not separated from the expiratory limb.

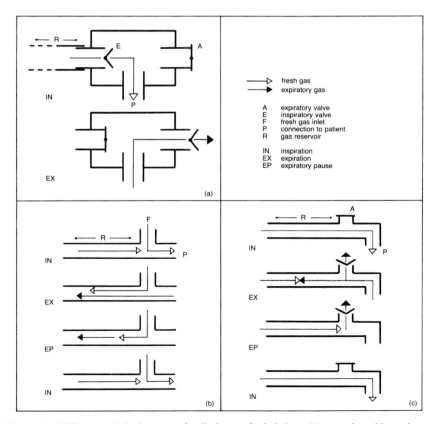

Figure 1.2   Different technical concepts for discharge of exhaled gas: (a) non-rebreathing valve (valve-controlled non-rebreathing system); (b) flow-controlled discharge of the exhaled gas via the reservoir tube (flow-controlled non-rebreathing system, type: Ayre's T-piece; (c) flow-controlled discharge of the exhaled gas via an expiratory valve (flow-controlled non-rebreathing system, type: Mapleson A)

Where the Ayre's T-piece, the Mapleson systems types D and E, the Kuhn, Jackson–Rees and the Bain systems are concerned, the expired gas is washed out of the system during the expiratory phase by a vigorous undirectional flow of fresh gas (Figure 1.2b).

However, with non-rebreathing systems of the Mapleson A (the Lack and Magill systems), B and C types, a vigorous fresh gas flow opposes the expiratory flow. Thus, during exhalation the pressure within the system increases which in turn opens an expiratory valve, through which the expiratory volume escapes from the system (Figure 1.2c).

Should the fresh gas flow not be sufficiently high, elimination of exhaled gas will be incomplete in all flow-controlled non-rebreathing systems. In principle, depending on the basic technical design of all flow-controlled non-rebreathing systems, rebreathing of exhaled gas is possible. Considerable rebreathing, however, will cause an undesirable carbon dioxide enrichment in the system due to the lack of a carbon dioxide absorber. It is for this reason that obligatory statements are made on the fresh gas flow for each of the systems in question to safely preclude excessive rebreathing (Table 1.1). In addition, the efficiency of eliminating expired gas at a defined fresh gas flow is influenced by the geometry and design of the system, the tidal and minute volume and the ventilatory pattern[3,6].

1.1.3   Systems without gas reservoir

Systems without reservoir are no longer used in present-day clinical routine and they differ greatly in respect of their technical design. This term covers a wide range of equipment such as drip anaesthetic masks and insufflation blades. However, the lack of a fresh gas reservoir enables an uncontrolled inspiratory admission of atmospheric air into all of these systems[6].

Table 1.1   Flow-controlled non-rebreathing systems – recommended fresh gas flows for prevention of excessive rebreathing (From References 1, 6, 9, 11–14)

	Spontaneous breathing	Controlled ventilation
Mapleson A Magill system Lack system	0.7–1 × MV	2–3 × MV
Mapleson B and C	2 × MV	2 × MV
Ayre T-piece Mapleson E Kuhn system	2 × MV	2–3 × MV
Jackson–Rees system	1.5 × MV	1–2 × MV
Mapleson D	1.5 × MV	1 × MV
Bain system	200–300 ml/min × kg	70 ml/min × kg
Humphrey–ADE system	> 50 ml/min × kg	> 70 ml/min × kg

MV, minute volume; kg, kilogram bodyweight.

1.2   Classification of breathing systems in accordance with functional criteria

1.2.1   Closed systems

A breathing system is referred to as being closed if the fresh gas volume that is fed into the system corresponds exactly to the uptake, i.e. the volume of gas which the patient takes up during the respective period of time. Following elimination of carbon dioxide, the entire expiratory gas volume is routed back to the patient in the following inspiratory phase. A sufficient gas volume within the system can only be maintained if the excess gas discharge valve is closed and the system is absolutely gas tight. We refer to 'quantitative anaesthesia with closed system' only if the composition and the volume of the fresh gas correspond at any time exactly to that amount of oxygen, nitrous oxide and volatile anaesthetic which is actually taken up by the patient[15]. However, if only the volume and not the composition of the fresh gas corresponds to the uptake of the patient, this is referred to as 'non-quantitative anaesthesia with closed system'.

1.2.2   Semi-closed systems

In the semi-closed system, the fresh gas flow fed into the breathing system is greater than the uptake, but less than the minute volume. This technique of anaesthetic management is only possible provided that the exhaled gas is partially rebreathed, but at the same time, excess gas escapes from the system. The recirculating gas volume is in inverse proportion to the fresh gas flow and the excess gas volume.

1.2.3   Semi-open systems

In the semi-open system, the exhaled gas is completely discharged out of the system, while pure fresh gas is administered to the patient during the following inspiration. This means, depending on the system's design, that the fresh gas flow must be at least equal to or many times above the minute volume. The amount of oxygen, nitrous oxide and volatile anaesthetic escaping from the system unused is proportional to the fresh gas flow.

1.2.4   Open systems

Open systems have one characteristic in common: precise control of the anaesthetic gas composition inhaled by the patient is not possible. The fact that a sufficient fresh gas reservoir is not available may, as a function of the tidal volume, result in an uncontrolled entrance of ambient air, or in uncontrollable changes in anaesthetic gas concentrations.

1.3   Breathing systems according to technical and functional aspects (Table 1.2)

1.3.1   Rebreathing systems

In terms of the basic technical concept, these systems are especially designed for rebreathing. They are used as closed systems if the fresh gas volume

Table 1.2   Breathing systems according to technical and functional aspects

	Open	Semi-open	Semi-closed	Closed
Rebreathing systems	∅	+	+	+
Flow-controlled non-breathing systems	(+)	+	(+)	∅
Valve-controlled non-rebreathing systems	(+)	+	∅	∅
Systems without reservoir	+	(+)	∅	∅

↔, adequate use; (+). unsafe limits of utilization; ∅, utilization mode incompatible with the technical concept.

corresponds to the uptake and, following carbon dioxide absorption, the exhaled gas is completely rebreathed by the patient.

With respect to function, they are semi-closed systems if the fresh gas flow is greater than the uptake, but less than the minute volume, and rebreathing is partial. Inevitably, the rebreathing volume decreases with increasing fresh gas flow, while the excess gas volume increases.

Given favourable design of the system – a circle system with the exhaust valve proximal to the expiratory limb and the fresh gas inlet being proximal to the inspiratory limb – plus a fresh gas flow that is greater than the alveolar ventilation volume, the rebreathing proportion is reduced to a negligible minimum[1]. The composition of the inspiratory gas is then virtually identical to the fresh gas, so that the rebreathing system functions as a semi-open system.

In terms of function, rebreathing systems cannot be open systems, since the closed design of these systems renders the free entrance of air impossible.

1.3.2   Non-rebreathing systems

1.3.2.1   Flow-controlled non-rebreathing systems

With respect to the basic technical concept, non-rebreathing systems are not designed for rebreathing, but for elimination of the exhaled gas, and inspiratory supply of fresh gas. Essentially, the efficiency of elimination of the expiratory gas depends on the technical design of the system, the tidal and minute volume and the breathing ventilation[6,16]. Accordingly, precise specifications are given for the different systems, as to the fresh gas flow which has to be selected to reliably prevent rebreathing, for both spontaneous breathing and controlled ventilation (see Table 1.1). These recommendations are always made with respect to the minute volume. To obtain the best efficiency of these systems, the fresh gas volume should be at least equal to the minute volume, in order to eliminate the entire expiratory volume. Thus, flow-controlled non-rebreathing systems are designed to be used as semi-open systems.

Should a lower fresh gas flow – 70% of the minute volume – be quoted for a particular system, this results in partial rebreathing without carbon dioxide absorption which can only be acceptable provided that this will not cause a considerable carbon dioxide enrichment. The rebreathed gas should be the dead space volume and not the carbon dioxide containing alveolar ventilation volume[1]. This results in a floating, but rather limited transition to a semi-closed use of flow-controlled non-rebreathing systems.

If the reservoir volume of the system is comparatively large, increasing reduction of the fresh gas flow causes a drastic rise in carbon dioxide concentration. If, on the other hand, the reservoir volume is comparatively small, air may be drawn into the system during inspiration, which in turn results in a functionally open system.

1.3.2.2   Valve-controlled non-rebreathing systems

Where valve-controlled non-rebreathing systems are concerned, rebreathing of the expiratory gas, which necessarily escapes via the non-rebreathing valve, is not possible. These systems cannot be used as closed or semi-closed systems. Since the inspiratory gas reliably consists of pure fresh gas, its flow must equal the minute volume. A further increase of fresh gas flow is unreasonable, since the resultant positive pressure in the inspiratory limb will impair the valve function, causing excess gas to be immediately discharged from the system via the expiratory valve. Thus valve-controlled non-rebreathing systems are used exclusively as semi-open systems.

Transition to the open system may be possible only if the inspiratory limb is open to the atmosphere, while the volume of the gas reservoir is too small or the fresh gas flow too low. Ambient air may thus be drawn into the system during inspiration.

1.3.3   Systems without gas reservoir

In this context, reference is made to the Boyle–Davis gag as an example. If the fresh gas flow is low, ambient air is inhaled in addition to the anaesthetic gas with every inspiration. By definition, this is an open system. If however, the fresh gas flow is high and the tidal volume low, the oropharynx, which is filled with fresh gas in the expiratory pause, acts as a fresh gas reservoir, so that the patient inhales fresh gas only. This represents a floating transition from the open to the semi-open system.

As a rule, it may be possible that all the different breathing systems assume the characteristics of an open system whenever ambient air can enter the system freely, and the entire volume of the fresh gas flow and the reservoir is lower than the inspiratory volume.

1.4   Function of breathing systems in relation to the fresh gas flow (Table 1.3)

In summary, breathing systems must be understood as being the technical elements which, as a function of the fresh gas flow selected, prepare the gas mixture which the patient inhales in a dynamic process from fresh gas, exhaled gas and, perhaps, ambient air. Thus they are not only components which passively administer the fresh gas to the patient prepared by the flow control system, the mixer and the vaporizer, but they are the elements by which the composition of the anaesthetic gases is determined.

Table 1.3   Function mode of different breathing systems in relation to the fresh gas flow, minute volume, and uptake

	Semi-open	Semi-closed	Closed
Rebreathing systems	FGF ⩾ MV	FGF > UPTAKE	FGF = UPTAKE
		FGF < MV	
Flow-controlled non-rebreathing systems	FGF ≫ MV	FGF ≈ MV	
Valve-controlled non-rebreathing systems	FGF = MV		

FGF, fresh gas flow; MV, minute volume.

Finally it is the method of anaesthesia management, which itself depends greatly on the selection of the fresh gas flow, that determines the function and dosage characteristics of the breathing system.

1.5   References

1. Ernst, E. A. Closed circuit anesthesia. In *Refresher-Kurs ZAK 85* (eds F. W. List and H. V. Schalk), Akademische Druck- und Verlagsanstalt, Graz (1985)
2. International Organisation for Standards (ISO): *ISO 4135:199X*, Revision of *ISO 4135:1979 – Anaesthesiology – Vocabulary*, British Standards Institution (1993)
3. Barth, L. and Meyer, M. *Moderne Narkose*, Fischer, Stuttgart (1965)
4. Dick, W., Altemeyer, K. H. and Schöch, G. Das Paedi-System. Ein neues Narkosesystem für Säuglinge und Kinder. *Anaesthesist*, **26** 369–371 (1977)
5. Dudziak, R. *Lehrbuch der Anästhesiologie*, Schattauer, Stuttgart (1980)
6 Gray, T. C., Nunn, J. F. and Utting, J. E. *General Anaesthesia*, Butterworth, London (1980)
7. Herden, H.-N. and Lawin, P. *Anästhesie-Fibel*, Thieme, Stuttgart (1973)
8. Larsen, R., Sonntag, H. and Kettler, D. *Anästhesie und Intensivmedizin für Schwestern und Pfleger*, Springer, Berlin (1984)
9. Lee, J. A. and Atkinson, R. S. *A Synopsis of Anaesthesia*, 7th edn, John Wright, Bristol (1973)
10. Davey, A., Moyle, J. T. B. and Ward, C. S. *Ward's Anaesthetic Equipment*, 3rd edn, W. B. Saunders, London (1992)
11 Bergmann, H. Das Narkosegerät in Gegenwart und Zukunft aus der Sicht des Klinikers. *Anaesthesist*, **35**, 587–594 (1986)
12. Humphrey, D. A new anaesthetic breathing system combining Mapleson A, D and E principles. *Anaesthesia*, **38**, 361–372 (1983)
13. Humphrey, D., Brock-Utne, J. G. and Downing, J. W. Multipurpose anaesthetic breathing systems – an update. In *Beiträge zur Anästhesiologie und Intensivmedizin*, Bd. 17 (eds H. Bergmann, H. Kramar and K. Steinbereithner), Maudrich, Wien (1986), p. 51
14. Lowe, H. J. and Ernst, E. A. *The Quantitative Practice of Anesthesia*, Williams and Wilkins, Baltimore (1981)
15. Baum, J. Clinical applications of low flow and closed circuit anesthesia. *Acta Anaesth. Belg.*, **41** 239–247 (1990)
16. Nemes, C., Niemer, M. and Noack, G. *Datenbuch Anästhesiologie*, Fischer, Stuttgart (1979)
17. Baum, J. Narkosesysteme. *Anaesthesist*, **36**, 393–399 (1987)

Rebreathing systems – the development of a technical concept

2.1 Development of breathing systems – historical perspective

The manifold possibilities and variants of inhalational anaesthesia are closely related to the technical development of anaesthetic machines. Competent evaluation of the advantages and disadvantages of rebreathing techniques, as well as the prejudices with regard to this technique, require such a background knowledge. The following brief and thus incomplete description of the development in technology of anaesthetic machines and breathing systems is based essentially on a number of textbooks[1-4] – as well as on some specialist publications on this topic[5-9].

2.1.1 Development of open systems

The first inhalational anaesthetic was performed by Crawford W. Long (1815–1880) on 3 March 1842 with ether. One of the first chloroform anaesthetics to be published was performed by James Y. Simpson (1811–1870) on 5 November 1847. Both physicians used a cloth soaked with the volatile anaesthetic, held over the mouth and nose of the patient[8,10,11]. The vapours were inhaled by the patient and put him into a narcotic sleep. This very simple method of inhalational anaesthesia was soon widely used. In 1862, Skinner developed something like a mask, a wire frame, into which the cloth was inserted. It was held in front of the patient's face so that skin and mucous tissues were protected from the liquid anaesthetic, while at the same time the narcotizing vapours could be more precisely applied and the cloth secured in place[8]. This concept was varied and improved in many ways, for example by Esmarch, Kocher and Schimmelbusch. Anaesthesia with these kinds of masks which, in technical terms are systems without gas reservoir, is nowadays rarely performed in developed countries.

These breathing systems do, however, feature a number of obvious advantages:

- minimal apparatus requirements
- uncomplicated method of anaesthetic application
- low respiratory resistance
- the use of this system is possible even under the most adverse infrastructural conditions.

Its disadvantages are quoted as follows:

- unexpected, non-controllable changes in anaesthetic depth resulting from uncontrollable changes of applied anaesthetic concentration
- considerable pollution of the operating theatre with anaesthetic vapours
- the resultant risk of fire and explosions.

2.1.2   Development of non-rebreathing systems

2.1.2.1   Valve-controlled non-rebreathing systems

The development of valve-controlled non-rebreathing systems is also closely related to the spread of ether anaesthesia. On 16 October 1846, William T. G. Morton (1819–1868) succeeded in demonstrating the first clinical ether anaesthetic[11] at the Massachusetts General Hospital in Boston. He used a special apparatus[8,12]; this Morton Ether Inhalator was the very first anaesthetic system (Figure 2.1). The Morton apparatus was a glass ball with two necks, which contained a sponge soaked with ether. One neck was fitted with a hose and a mouthpiece through which the patient inhaled the ether vapours. The ambient air which entered the glass ball through the other neck promoted the ether evaporation process. Exhalation took place through the mouthpiece, back into the inhalation system. It was during this first clinical demonstration that Morton realized that the patient's exhalation into the system was disadvantageous. The system used on the following day and described by H. J. Bigelow[13], was therefore fitted with a valve close to the mouthpiece, allowing exhaled air to escape into the atmosphere.

An improvement of this technical concept was the breathing system designed by John Snow (1813–1858). His apparatus was equipped with a generously dimensioned breathing hose, an inspiratory and expiratory valve and a more precisely working ether vaporizer. The advantages of this system were a reduced respiratory resistance and the possibility of more accurate dosage of the ether vapour. Further development of this concept in 1941 by Prof. Macintosh and Dr Epstein led to the Oxford Vaporizer, the breathing system of which was fitted with a non-rebreathing valve in proximity to the patient's airway[8].

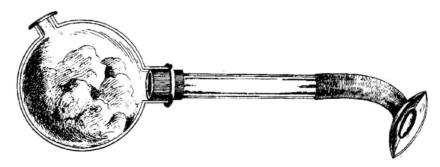

Figure 2.1   Dieffenbach's modification of Morton's apparatus for ether inhalation (From Dieffenbach[12])

Such valve-controlled non-rebreathing systems with precisely operating vaporizers are still manufactured and used nowadays, as is reflected for instance in the AFYA anaesthesia machine of the Dräger company, Lübeck.

2.1.2.2   Flow-controlled non-rebreathing systems

The development of flow-controlled non-rebreathing systems is closely related to the use of nitrous oxide as an anaesthetic gas. Humphry Davy (1778–1829) discussed the possibility of eliminating pain in surgical interventions with the aid of nitrous oxide as early as 1800: 'As nitrous oxide in its extensive operation appears capable of destroying physical pain, it may probably be used with advantage during surgical operations in which no great effusion of blood takes place'[14]. Following a successful self-test on 11 December 1844, Horace Wells (1815–1848) performed the first clinical demonstration of nitrous oxide as an inhalational anaesthetic at the Massachusetts General Hospital in Boston, in January 1845[10,15]. However, this demonstration was not successful and Davy's idea of inhibiting pain by means of nitrous oxide was dismissed by the surgeon Warren as being charlatanry and swindle. Some 18 years later, Gardner Q. Colton (1814–1898) made another attempt to arouse interest in this inhalational anaesthetic. But with his method of administration, patients inhaled pure nitrous oxide from a breathing bag up to the state of asphyxia, the effect was not obtained reliably and was too brief for longer surgical procedures. In 1868, E. Andrews (1824–1904) was the first to recommend the use of an oxygen–nitrous oxide mixture, for safe anaesthesia even in longer lasting operations[16].

The development of anaesthesia machines (H. Th. Hillischer, 1886; F. W. Hewitt, 1893), by means of which the the patient could be supplied with an oxygen–nitrous oxide mixture of defined composition, was a decisive step forward in this direction. In addition, cylinders with pressure regulators were used as oxygen and nitrous oxide reservoirs, which made anaesthetics available at a high continuous flow[8]. M. Neu introduced an apparatus in 1910, permitting accurate adjustment of nitrous oxide and oxygen flows by means of precision needle valves, which could be measured with the aid of flowmeter tubes[17]. This measurement and dosing principle is still applied in the most advanced present-day machines. From then on it was possible to maintain anaesthesia over lengthy periods without the danger of hypoxia. However, exhaled gas had to be discharged into the atmosphere after each breath via an exhaust valve, since the technique of carbon dioxide absorption was not available in those times. Great volumes of expensive anaesthetic gases, which were very scarce, were inevitably lost.

The construction of the different flow-controlled breathing systems, which are still used today, is based on the development of anaesthetic machines which permit the administration of a defined anaesthetic gas mixture at a high constant flow. These are, for instance, the Ayre's T-piece and the Bain, Kuhn, Lack and Magill systems. A gas mixture consisting of oxygen, nitrous oxide and a volatile anaesthetic agent is administered to the patient. The gas flow must be tuned to the breathing or ventilation parameters of the patient and to the design of the system in order that rebreathing can be precluded. The technical concept of flow-controlled non-rebreathing systems thus requires a constant gas flow at a high rate.

The advantages of non-rebreathing systems are:

- the composition of anaesthetic gas corresponds to the fresh gas
- easy control of the anaesthetic concentration by direct variation of the fresh gas composition
- comparatively few technical requirements.

The disadvantages which have to be taken into consideration are:

- high consumption of anaesthetic agents
- excessive pollution with anaesthetic gases
- low temperature and humidity of the respired gases.

2.1.3   Development of rebreathing systems

As early as in 1850 – only 4 years after the first successful clinical performance of ether anaesthesia – John Snow (1813–1858) recognized that ether and chloroform were exhaled unchanged with the expired air. To reuse these unchanged vapours in the following inspiration and thereby prolonging the narcotic effect of a given amount of anaesthetic vapour, he converted his ether inhaler (Figure 2.2) into a to-and-fro rebreathing system. The apparatus was equipped with a face mask, without inspiratory or expiratory valves, and a large reservoir bag containing pure oxygen attached to the air inlet; the spiral chamber was filled partially with an aqueous solution of caustic potash which was used as a carbon dioxide absorbent. In several experiments, performed on himself, Snow succeeded in demonstrating that rebreathing of the exhaled vapours was possible following carbon dioxide absorption, and

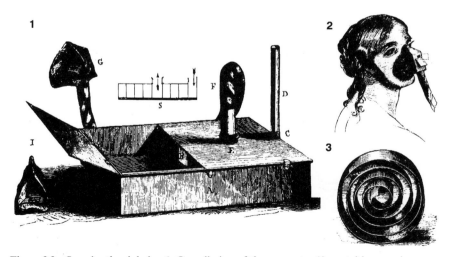

Figure 2.2   Snow's ether inhaler. 1. Overall view of the apparatus (A, metal box serving as a water bath; B, spiral ether chamber; C, opening for filling in ether; D, brass tube by which the air enters which the patient inhales; E, outlet of the ether chamber; F, elastic tube; G, face piece; I, the same face piece compressed, to fit it to a smaller face; S, section of spiral ether chamber). 2. Face piece with inspiratory and expiratory valve. 3. Ether chamber with the bottom removed, showing the volute (From Snow[22])

that it resulted in a pronounced prolongation of the narcotic effects of the volatile anaesthetics[18]. Furthermore, Snow performed experiments on animals using a closed system (Figure 2.3) for evaluating the carbon dioxide production during anaesthesia[19,20].

Yet the principle of rebreathing exhaled air via a breathing system after elimination of 'noxious vapours' had long since been known[7]. In 1727, Stephen Hales (1677–1761) described a rebreathing circle system by means of which 'sulphureous steams' could be absorbed, destroying the 'elasticity of the air' and thus rendering impossible free ventilation[21]. His breathing system, which he recommended for rescue purposes, consisted of a gas reservoir made of a bladder into which four diaphragms of flannel were placed, soaked with a solution of highly calcinated tartar, a wide-bore siphon, and unidirectional inspiratory and expiratory valves (Figure 2.4).

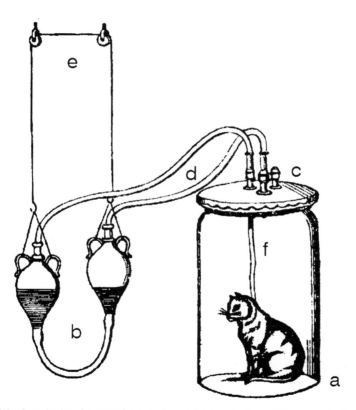

Figure 2.3 Snow's closed system for experimental determination of the amount of carbon dioxide excreted during ether and chloroform anaesthesia. a, Glass jar; b, two glass vessels, filled with an aqueous solution of potash, connected together by an elastic tube; c, airtight lid with an opening for filling in the volatile anaesthetic; d, rubber tubes connecting the jar with the potash apparatus; e, mechanism to move up and down the glass vessels. If the glass vessels were moved up and down they alternately filled with the fluid, resulting in a constant circulation of the air within the jar and the vessels and, thus, leading to absorption of the exhaled carbon dioxide by the solution of potash (From Snow[20])

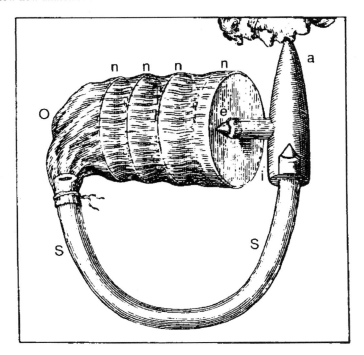

Figure 2.4   Hale's closed rebreathing system of 1727. a, Mouthpiece; e, unidirectional expiratory valve; i, unidirectional inspiratory valve; n, four linen diaphragms clamped into the breathing gas reservoir, soaked with calcinated potassium bitartrate for carbon dioxide absorption; o, flexible breathing gas reservoir; s, inspiratory hose (From Rendell-Baker[7], by permission)

A mine rescue apparatus from Schwann, which featured a high pressure oxygen reservoir cylinder, reducing and flow control valves plus circle breathing system with carbon dioxide absorber, was already available in 1856[7].

Alfred Coleman (1828–1902) was the first to use a to-and-fro system with carbon dioxide absorption in clinical practice (Figure 2.5). Nitrous oxide was delivered to a pair of reservoir bags connected together with a unidirectional valve. From the proximal reservoir the patient inhaled the gas, which had to pass a tin box filled with slaked lime, via a wide-bore tubing leading to a face mask. During expiration the air was expired back into the proximal reservoir bag, again passing the metal box where the carbon dioxide was absorbed. By the use of rebreathing technique, Coleman wanted to decrease nitrous oxide consumption, as the usual use of high amounts of this expensive anaesthetic was a serious impediment to the spread of nitrous oxide anaesthesia. As the patients got pure nitrous oxide, this rebreathing technique could only be used in very short surgical procedures. Although Coleman committedly advocated the use of his 'economising apparatus', this technique was not generally adopted[23].

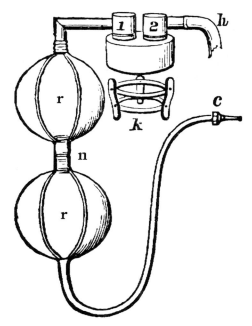

Figure 2.5   Coleman's 'economising apparatus'. c, Adapter to the nitrous oxide cylinder; r, reservoir bags; n, unidirectional valve; 1 and 2, metal box (economiser), filled with small pieces of slaked lime; 1, connector to the reservoir bags; 2, connector to the patient; h, tubing to the face piece; k, frame which supports the economiser on the top of the gas cylinder (From Duncum[23], by permission)

In 1906, Franz Kuhn (1866–1929) published the constructive details of a concept for a breathing system which incorporated a similar technical component for elimination of carbon dioxide from the exhaled gas (Figure 2.6). It was also Kuhn's intention to lead back unused anaesthetic gases, contained in the expired air, to the patient during the following inhalation. The amount of oxygen to be fed into the system then merely had to replenish the volume which had been consumed or got lost as a result of leaks. However, this system was never put to clinical use since the flow resistance and the dead space of the breathing system were too great. In addition, Kuhn feared that the chemical reaction of chloroform with the absorbing material (caustic soda) might possibly harm the patient[41].

In 1915, Dennis E. Jackson (1879–1980) reported prolonged anaesthesia in animals by means of a closed circle system with carbon dioxide absorption (Figure 2.7), using a gas mixture of volatile anaesthetics, nitrous oxide and oxygen[24]. Neither the apparatus nor the method met with any interest, although the use of this technology saved considerable amounts of anaesthetic gas and the apparatus itself worked reliably. In 1916, Jackson described a very simple and cheap to-and-fro system for experimental anaesthesia[25], in which a cake pan, partially filled with an aqueous solution of soda lime, was used for absorption of the exhaled carbon dioxide (Figure 2.8).

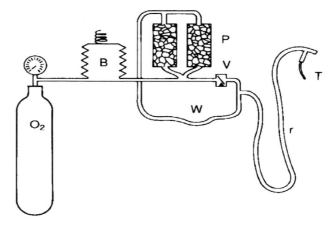

Figure 2.6 Concept of a rebreathing system developed by Franz Kuhn (in 1906). B, bellows; P, carbon dioxide absorber; V, inspiratory valve; W, breathing system; T, airway; r, breathing tube (From Rendell-Baker[7], by permission)

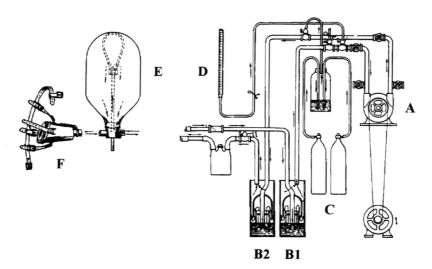

Figure 2.7 Jackson's circle absorption system. The animal inhales gas via a face piece (F) out of a rubber bag which serves as a gas reservoir (E). Anaesthetic gas is continuously sucked out of this reservoir by an air pump (A). The gas passes the wash jar (B1), filled with concentrated sulphuric acid, leaves the pump in the direction of the wash jar (B2), filled with a strong aqueous solution of sodium hydrate and calcium hydrate, passes a Woulff bottle and is then returned back to the gas reservoir. Nitrous oxide and oxygen, obtained from the gas cylinders (C), are fed into the system in just such an amount to keep constant the filling level of the gas reservoir. Fluid ether or chloroform is delivered into the system from the burette (D). (From Jackson[24])

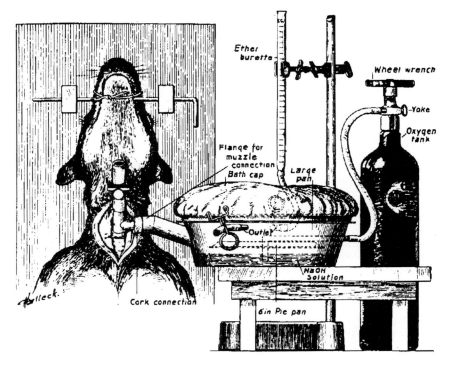

Figure 2.8 Jackson's to-and-fro absorption system. Very simple to-and-fro system built from parts bought in a ten cent store: the absorber, simultaneously serving as a vaporizer and a gas reservoir, consists of a cake and a pie pan and a bath cap (From Jackson[25])

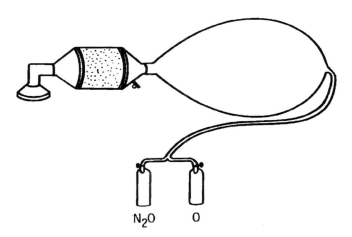

Figure 2.9 The to-and-fro system of R. M. Waters (From Waters[26])

It was Ralph M. Waters (1883–1979) who introduced the technique of anaesthesia with closed rebreathing system into medical practice in 1924[26]. In his to-and-fro system, it was a metal canister filled with sodium hydroxide granules which served as a carbon dioxide absorber (Figure 2.9). The patient inhaled anaesthetic gas from the reservoir bag into which he exhaled again. Adequate oxygenation was achieved by intermittent oxygen supply. Hans Killian paid a visit to Waters in Madison (USA) in 1928 and was greatly impressed by his work with the to-and-fro system[27]:

> ... After the patient had been slightly anaesthetised in an anteroom, he [Waters] filled a large 10-litre balloon with an ethylene and oxygen mixture from the Foregger machine, at a ratio of about 80:20%. Then he switched off the machine completely, closed the filling tap of the large rubber bag, attached a soda cartridge to it, and to the other end fitted an anaesthetic mask, which was placed onto the patient's face. The patient inhaled the gas mixture from the rubber bag only and expired back into the balloon. This was in accordance with his to-and-fro system and absorption of carbon dioxide. ... He [the patient] remained sleeping, although he did not receive a continuous flow of fresh gas, ethylene–oxygen. This balloon technique did not appear surprising as long as it lasted only 5 to 10 minutes for transport from the induction room to the operating theatre. But in this case it lasted much longer, 20 to 30 minutes. I noticed that Waters administered oxygen without ethylene into the bag only once, when the patient turned slightly blue. I was somewhat puzzled. Right in front of our eyes, a most remarkable event had taken place, much to my amazement. Though most of the others had not noticed it. Waters had proved that there was something wrong about our pharmacological assumptions that maintenance of the depth of sleep solely depends on the concentration of the inhalational anaesthetic. ... One can hardly imagine how this whole story embarrassed me. I lay awake late the following night, thinking and trying with all my might to get behind the secret and to come up with an idea about our anaesthetic methods. ... We were really on the verge of an outstanding progress in the field of anaesthesia. ...

Rebreathing systems were also developed in Germany between 1920 and 1924. First Carl J. Gauss (1875–1957) at the University of Göttingen[28] and, one year later, Paul Sudeck and Helmut Schmidt from the University Hospital Hamburg-Eppendorf[29] performed anaesthesia with breathing systems in which the exhaled air circulated by valve control and, following blending with fresh anaesthetic gas, was routed back to the patient. Their systems incorporated carbon dioxide absorbers, and in terms of technical concept, these circle absorption systems were definitely rebreathing systems[9]. Based on the experience of these physicians, the Dräger company, Lübeck, manufactured the 'Lachgas-Narkose-Apparat Modell A nach Sudeck, Schmidt und Dräger' from 1925 onwards (Figure 2.10). Nitrous oxide and oxygen were obtained from cylinders via pressure regulators, and flowmeters permitted precise dosage of gas volumes to be fed into the circle system[5]. In the Anglo-American literature, however, development of the circle absorption system is ascribed to B. C. Sword (1889–1956)[30]. The majority of anaesthesia machines used today are equipped with such rebreathing circle absorption systems.

Essentially, the advantages of the rebreathing system[3,4] have already been summarized by Waters[26]:

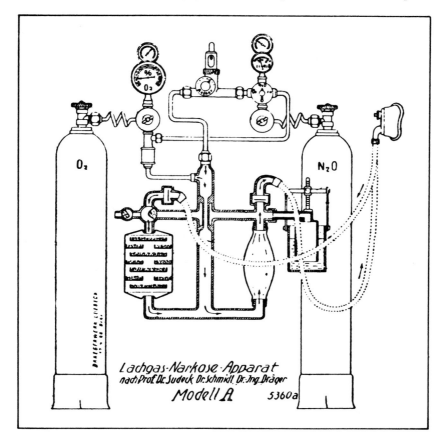

Figure 2.10   Flow diagram of the circle absorption system of the Dräger
Lachgas-Narkose-Apparat Modell A of 1925 (From Haupt[5], by permission)

- considerable savings in anaesthetic gases
- reduced contamination of the ambient atmosphere
- reduced danger of explosion in using explosive inhalation anaesthetics
- improved humidification and warming of the anaesthetic gases
- reduced loss of heat and moisture.

The following points are regarded as being disadvantageous[3,4]:

- technically involved systems with carbon dioxide absorbers
- reduced safety against oxygen deficiency
- increased possibility of unnoticed carbon dioxide rebreathing in case of soda lime exhaustion.

However, in evaluating rebreathing systems, Moser[4] comes to the conclusion that the advantages of anaesthesia management with these systems far outweighs the disadvantages.

2.2   Development of anaesthesia management with semi-closed rebreathing systems – considerations on the current situation

Anaesthesia management with closed or virtually closed rebreathing systems has gained increasing popularity since the technical tools for the rebreathing technique have been available[31]. This may also be attributed to the introduction of the flammable and indeed explosive cyclopropane as an anaesthetic agent in 1933[32]. Thanks to the consistent utilization of the rebreathing technique, the discharge of excess gas from the breathing system could be reduced, so that consequently the cyclopropane concentration in the operating theatre could be maintained at the lowest possible level.

With the increasing use of sodium thiopentone for rapid induction (1934) and curare (1942) for potent and safe muscle relaxation, the popularity of cyclopropane and the necessity to extensively reduce the excess gas discharge declined. Furthermore, the danger of unintended delivery of hypoxic gas mixtures when using rebreathing systems was recognized[32]. A broadsheet against the deliberate application of hypoxic anaesthetic gas mixtures was published by Barach and Rovenstine[33]. They recommended the use of a fixed oxygen nitrous oxide mixture (20% O_2, 80% N_2O), delivered with high flow, from a reservoir tank directly to the patient. This is why in German textbooks the use of fresh gas flows of about 4 l/min or even higher containing at least 25% oxygen was recommended as being safe[1,34].

The introduction of the volatile anaesthetic halothane in 1956 reinforced the tendency for considerable changes in anaesthesia management. From then on, the use of high fresh gas flows, that is anaesthesia management with a semi-closed system, has gained significant prominence.

The higher the fresh gas flow, the more the composition of the anaesthetic gas corresponded to the fresh gas (Figure 2.11). However, the higher the fresh gas flow, the greater was the volume of excess gas discharged from the system, and the lower the rebreathing volume. Rebreathing systems were, as a result, increasingly used without rebreathing. This development was supported by a number of factors[31,32,35]:

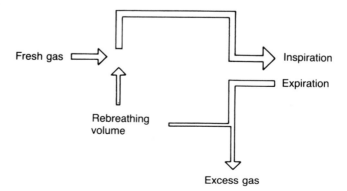

Figure 2.11   Schematic flow diagram of a semi-closed rebreathing circle system

1. At that time, the vaporizers available – TEC type or Copper Kettle (Figure 2.12) – did not allow precise dosage of halothane at low gas flows[36,37]: patients who were being ventilated suffered from perilous overdosage, on occasions with a fatal outcome.
2. There was great uncertainty with respect to the dose and pharmacokinetics of this highly efficient volatile anaesthetic which was characterized by an unusually low therapeutic index.
3. Observation of spontaneous breathing as a criterion for evaluation of anaesthetic depth was no longer relevant during controlled ventilation of an anaesthetized and relaxed patient. As an alternative, the depth of anaesthesia was now estimated in accordance with the minimum alveolar concentration (MAC) principle by means of the anaesthetic concentration applied. However, this was practicable only when the composition of anaesthetic gas corresponded approximately to that of the fresh gas.

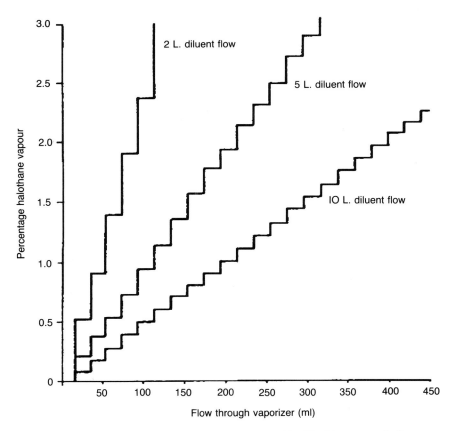

Figure 2.12 Changes in halothane concentration produced by 20 ml increments in flow through the copper kettle at 20°C, with different diluent (fresh gas) flows of 2, 5 and 10 litres per minute (From Feldman and Morris[36], by permission)

4. The increasing utilization of positive pressure ventilation was accompanied by increasing loss of gas from leaks and this could only be compensated for by an increase in the fresh gas flow.
5. The costs involved for oxygen and nitrous oxide could be considerably reduced by using central piping systems for medical gases.
6. The practical performance of anaesthesia with a high excess gas volume does not require knowledge of pharmacokinetic characteristics with respect to the uptake and distribution of volatile anaesthetics or a subtle understanding of apparatus functions. The interest in acquiring such knowledge decreased, which may be attributed to the fact that anaesthetists were taking over a great number of new tasks which occupied their attention during anaesthesia.
7. The problem of operating theatre contamination by large volumes of excess gas discharged from the systems seemed to be solved by use of activated charcoal filters and the installation of central anaesthetic gas scavenging systems. The unnecessary and possibly ecologically questionable contamination of the atmosphere by anaesthetic gases did not meet with any attention in those days.

Nowadays, preference is given to anaesthesia management with the semi-closed rebreathing system using a comparatively high fresh gas flow, presumably for medicolegal reasons. Accordingly, anaesthetists learn extremely little about specific problems, but also nothing about the special advantages of anaesthesia management with low fresh gas flows, during the course of their education. Essential knowledge, such as uptake and distribution characteristics of oxygen, nitrous oxide and volatile anaesthetics and the effect of fresh gas flow on the function of breathing systems, is no longer imparted. The great uncertainty with respect to the nomenclature of breathing systems[38] reflects the generally inadequate knowledge of equipment function. By becoming accustomed to excessive fresh gas flows, less attention is paid to daily equipment maintenance and leak testing. This also applies to technical inspections or the production of anaesthetic machines, since high leakage losses – more than 10 l/min has been quoted at a pressure within the system of $20 \, cm \, H_2O$ – are accepted which, of course, makes flow reduction impossible.

The absolutely incomprehensible contradiction between the high technical specifications placed on equipment that is especially designed for rebreathing (i.e. the draft of the common European Standard on anaesthetic machines prEN 740)[39], on the one hand, and daily anaesthetic practice on the other, in which high fresh gas flows are used which render rebreathing systems with carbon dioxide absorption almost dispensable, has been emphasized by Bergmann[40].

With the circle absorption system, the anaesthetist now has available a perfect, technically advanced and reliable rebreathing tool, which is well proven in daily practice. Mandatory stipulations on safety features of modern anaesthetic machines are entirely focused upon anaesthesia management with rebreathing systems. However, the advantages of this sophisticated equipment cannot be used to their full potential because of the general trend towards the use of high fresh gas flows. This is why Bergmann comes to the conclusion[40]:

And yet it seems reasonable that in view of today's technical potentials of continuous monitoring of breathing gases, the technical perfection of the system itself, and the importance which is attached to the gas tightness of the systems, and the accuracy of the flow control systems and vaporizers, all further efforts should be focused upon a sure return to the closed system.

2.3 References

1. Barth, L. and Meyer, M. *Moderne Narkose*, Fischer, Stuttgart (1965)
2. Killian, H. and Weese, H. *Die Narkose*, Thieme, Stuttgart (1954)
3. Minnitt, R. J. and Gillies, J. *Textbook of Anaesthetics*, 6th edn, E. & S. Livingstone, Edinburgh (1945)
4. Moser, H. Die Praxis der modernen Narkose. In *Wiener Beiträge zur Chirurgie*, Bd. VI (ed. R. Demel), Maudrich, Wien (1951)
5. Haupt, J. *Der Dräger-Narkoseapparat – historisch gesehen*, Sonderdruck MT 105, Drägerwerk AG, Lübeck (1983)
6. Just, O. H., Dressler, P., Böhrer, H. and Wiedemann, K. Zur Geschichte der Anästhesie an der Universität Heidelberg. *Anästh. Intensivther. Notfallmed.*, **21**, 53–59 (1986)
7. Rendell-Baker, L. History of thoracic anaesthesia. In *Thoracic Anaesthesia* (ed. W. W. Mushin), Blackwell Scientific Publications, Oxford (1963)
8. Thomas, K. B. *The Development of Anaesthetic Apparatus*, Blackwell Scientific Publications, Oxford (1980)
9. Wawersik, J. Entwicklung der Narkosegeräte. In *Anaesthesie – historisch gesehen* (Hrsg. K. Zinganell), Springer, Berlin (1987)
10. Colton, G. Q.* *Anaesthesia. Who Made and Developed the Great Discovery?* A. G. Sherwood & Co., New York (1886)
11. Knight, N. *Pain and its Relief*, Smithsonian Institution, Washington (1988)
12. Dieffenbach, J. F. Apparate zum Einatmen der Ätherdämpfe. In *Der Äther gegen den Schmerz*, Hirschwald, Berlin (1847)
13. Bigelow, H. J.* Insensibility during surgical operations produced by inhalation. *Boston Medical and Surgical Journal*, **35**, 309–317 (1846)
14. Davy, H.* *Researches, Chemical and Philosophical; Chiefly Concerning Nitrous Oxide, or Dephlogisticated Nitrous Air, and its Respiration*, printed for J. Johnson, London by Biggs and Cottle, Bristol (1800)
15. Wells, H.* *A History of the Discovery of the Application of Nitrous Oxide Gas, Ether, and other Vapors to Surgical Operations*, J. G. Wells, Hartford (1847)
16. Andrews, E.* The oxygen mixture, a new anaesthetic combination. *Chicago Medical Examiner*, **9**, 656–661 (1868)
17. Neu, M. Ein Verfahren zur Stickoxidulsauerstoffnarkose. *Münch. med. Wschr,* **57**, 1873 (1910)
18. Snow, J. On Narcotism by the Inhalation of Vapours. Part XV. The effects of Chloroform and Ether Prolonged by Causing the Exhaled Vapour to be reinspired. *London Medical Gazette*, **11**, 749–754 (1850)
19. Baum, J. John Snow (1813–1858): Experimentelle Untersuchungen zur Rückatmung der in der Ausatemluft enthaltenen Narkosegase. *Anästhesiol. Intensivmed. Notfallmed. Schmerzther.*, **30**, 37–41 (1995)
20. Snow, J. On Narcotism by the Inhalation of Vapours. Part XVI. Experiments to determine the amount of Carbonic Acid Gas excreted under the influence of Chloroform. *London Medical Gazette*, **12**, 622–627 (1851)
21. Hales, S. Analysis of the air. Experiment CXVI. In *Statical Essays: Containing Vegetable Staticks; Or, An Account of some Statical Experiments On The Sap in Vegetables & Also, A Specimen of an Attempt to Analyse the Air, by a great Variety of Chymio-Statical Experiments, which were Read at Several Meetings before the Royal Society*, Vol I, 2nd edn, W. Innys, London (1731), pp. 264–273

22. Snow, J. *On the Inhalation of the Vapour of Ether in Surgical Operations*, John Churchill, London (1847)
23. Duncum, B. M. *The Development of Inhalation Anaesthesia*, Oxford University Press, London (1947), reprint edited on behalf of the History of Anaesthesia Society by the Royal Society of Medicine Press, London (1994), pp. 287–289
24. Jackson, D. E.* A new method for the production of general analgesia and anaesthesia with a description of the apparatus used. *J. Lab. Clin. Med.*, **1**, 1–12 (1915)
25. Jackson, D. E. The employment of closed ether anesthesia for ordinary laboratory experiments. *J. Lab. Clin. Med.*, **2**, 94–102 (1916)
26. Waters, R. M.* Clinical scope and utility of carbon dioxide filtration in inhalation anaesthesia. Anesth. Analg., **3**, 20–22 (1924)
27. Killian, H. *40 Jahre Narkoseforschung*, Verlag der Deutschen Hochschullehrerzeitung, Tübingen (1964)
28. Gauss, C. J. Die Narcylenbetäubung mit dem Kreisatmer. *Zentralblatt für Gynäkologie* **23**, 1218–1226 (1925)
29. Schmidt, H. Über Stickoxidulnarkose. Technische Überlegungen und Erfahrungen. *Bruhns Beiträge Klin. Chir.*, **137**, 506–518 (1926)
30. Sword, B. C.* The closed circle method of administration of gas anesthesia. *Curr. Res. Anesth. Analg.* **9**, 198–202 (1930)
31. Lowe, H. J. and Ernst, E. A. *The Quantitative Practice of Anesthesia*, Williams and Wilkins, Baltimore (1979)
32. Onishchuk, J. L. The early history of low-flow anaesthesia. In *The History of Anesthesia* (eds B. R. Fink, L. E. Morris and C. R. Stephen), Third International Symposium, Proceedings, Wood Library-Museum of Anesthesiology, Park Ridge, Illinois (1992), pp. 308–313
33. Barach, A. L. and Rovenstine, E. A. The hazard of anoxia during nitrous oxide anesthesia. *Anesthesiology*, **6**, 449–461 (1945)
34. Herden, H. N. and Lawin, P. *Anästhesie Fibel*, Thieme, Stuttgart (1973)
35. Buijs, B. H. M. J. Herwaardering van het Gesloten Ademsysteem in de Anesthesiologie (Reevaluation of Closed Circuit Anaesthesia), Diss. der Erasmus-Universität, Rotterdam (1988)
36. Feldman, S. A. and Morris, L. E. Vaporization of halothane and ether in the copper kettle. *Anesthesiology*, **19**, 650–655 (1958)
37. Hill, D. W. and Lowe, H. J. Comparison of concentration of halothane in closed and semiclosed circuits during controlled ventilation. *Anesthesiology*, **23**, 291–298 (1962)
38. Baum, J. Narkosesysteme. *Anaesthesist*, **36**, 393–399 (1987)
39. European Committee for Standardization (CEN). *Anaesthetic Workstations and their Modules*, prEN 740: Rev. 6.0. Paris (1994)
40. Bergmann, H. Das Narkosegerät in Gegenwart und Zukunft aus der Sicht des Klinikers. *Anaesthesist*, **35**, 587–594 (1986)
41. Kuhn, F. Die perorale Intubation mit und oline Druck. III. Teil. Apparat fur hieferung des Drudees für die Überdrucknarkose. *Deut. Zeitschr. Chir.* **81**, 63–70 (1906)

* Source of supply for facsimile prints of these publications: Wood Library-Museum of Anesthesiology, 520 North Nordwest Highway, Park Ridge, Illinois 60068-2573, USA.

Pharmacokinetics of anaesthetic gases

3.1 Oxygen

3.1.1 Oxygen uptake and consumption

According to Brody[1], the oxygen consumption of all homoiotherms can be calculated as an exponential function of the body weight in kilograms (BW(kg)), according to the formula:

$$\dot{V}_{O_2} = 10.15 \times BW(kg)^{0.73} \, (ml/min)$$

Kleiber[2] quoted a simplified formula for calculation of oxygen consumption at resting conditions, which is now generally known as the Brody formula:

$$\dot{V}_{O_2} = 10 \times BW(kg)^{3/4} \, (ml/min)$$

If the shape of the curve calculated by means of the Brody equation is approximated by two straight lines of different gradients, the oxygen consumption of two groups of different weight can be even more easily calculated[3]:

for body weight between 10 and 40 kg:

$$\dot{V}_{O_2} = 3.75 \times BW(kg) + 20 \, (ml/min)$$

for body weight between 40 and 120 kg:

$$\dot{V}_{O_2} = 2.5 \times BW(kg) + 67.5 \, (ml/min)$$

Not only is the oxygen consumption (Figure 3.1) correlated with the body weight raised to the power of 3/4 (BW (kg)$^{3/4}$), but also the carbon dioxide production, the alveolar ventilation and the cardiax output[2,4-6]. According to H. Lowe, the oxygen consumption decreases during induction of anaesthesia by about 15–30% with respect to the initial preoperative value[6]. Arndt[4] could demonstrate, by his investigations, that during anaesthesia oxygen consumption virtually corresponds to the basal metabolic rate. During anaesthesia, the oxygen consumption may be influenced by a great number of different factors: with decrease in temperature by 1°C, it falls by about 10%, and in case of acidosis by about 6% per 0.1 pH change. Certain anaesthetic agents such as ether, ketamine and etomidate increase the $\dot{V}_{O_2}$, just as does a respiratory or metabolic alkalosis[4]. In addition, the $\dot{V}_{O_2}$ is subject to variations with anaesthetic depth and the degree of relaxation

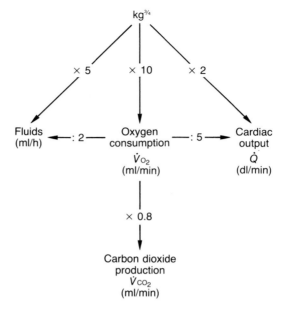

Figure 3.1   Calculation of physiological figures in relation to the body weight $(BW(kg)^{3/4})$ (From Lowe and Ernst[6], by permission)

within a range of about 10–25%[7,8]. Changes in cardiac output will also result in alterations of the oxygen uptake. Manawadu *et al.*[9] showed in animal experiments that a blood loss of 30% decreases the oxygen uptake by $30 \pm 10\%$ with respect to the initial value. Furthermore, oxygen consumption is reduced with age, which must be attributed to the reduction of metabolically active muscle mass in favour of fat and connective tissue[6].

Nevertheless it is justified to assume that the oxygen uptake during anaesthesia, which represents the oxygen consumption, remains comparatively constant in case of stable circulatory conditions, so that it can be calculated by means of the Brody formula with adequate accuracy (Figure 3.2).

3.1.2   Implications for anaesthetic practice

Any general anaesthetic results in a reduction of pulmonary function, irrespective of the anaesthetic method employed, the ventilation pattern and the duration. The alveolar–arterial oxygen partial pressure difference $(P_{(A-a)}O_2)$ and the intrapulmonary shunt will increase, while the functional residual capacity and the compliance of the lung will decrease. These changes are more pronounced in the elderly and obese than in the young and leptosome patients[10,11].

In order to prevent hypoxaemia reliably and to ensure continuous and sufficient oxygen supply, the inspired oxygen concentration should amount to at least 30%[12].

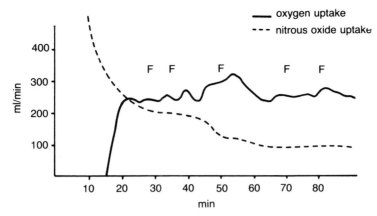

Figure 3.2   Nitrous oxide and oxygen uptake, measured during quantitative closed system anaesthesia with the aid of electronic control of gas dosage by closed-loop feedback. Steady-state conditions are not attained before denitrogenation is completed, approximately 25 min after induction of anaesthesia (F, i.v. administration of 0.05 mg fentanyl) (From Westenskow et al.[7], by permission)

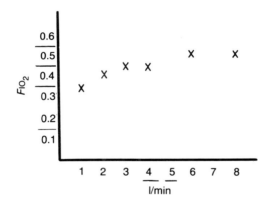

Figure 3.3   With constant fresh gas composition (50% O_2, 50% N_2O), the inspired oxygen concentration (y-axis) decreases with reduction of the fresh gas volume (x-axis) (From Schilling and Weis[13], by permission)

Fresh gas flow and fresh gas composition have a considerable effect on the oxygen concentration of inspired gas if anaesthesia is performed with a rebreathing circle system. Therefore, the following must be considered if the fresh gas flow is changed:

• up to a fresh gas flow of 10 l/min, the oxygen concentration in the inspiratory limb of a circle system will always be lower than that of the fresh gas[13]

• given a constant fresh gas composition (50% O_2 in Figure 3.3), the inspired oxygen concentration will drop once the flow is reduced (Figure 3.3)

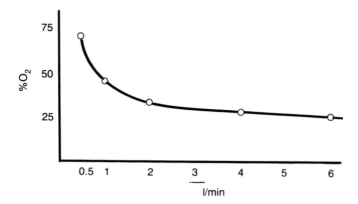

Figure 3.4   To ensure a constant oxygen concentration of 25% by volume, the oxygen content of the fresh gas (*y*-axis) must be increased if the fresh gas volume (*x*-axis) is reduced (From Schreiber[14], by permission)

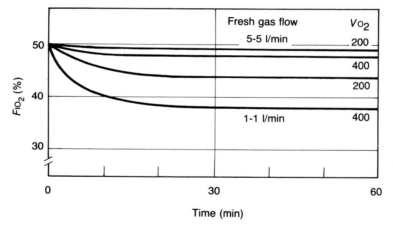

Figure 3.5   If the oxygen consumption ($\dot{V}_{O_2}$) rises to 400 ml/min, a low fresh gas flow (1 l/min $O_2 + 1$ l/min N_2O) results in a distinctly greater reduction of the inspired oxygen concentration (*y*-axis) than a high flow (5 l/min $O_2 + 5$ l/min N_2O) (From Westenskow[15], by permission)

● this means that, when the fresh gas volume is reduced, its oxygen content must be increased to ensure a constant oxygen concentration in the inspired gas (25% O_2 in Figure 3.4).

The proportion of exhaled gas in the inspired gas increases at low fresh gas flows. An increased oxygen consumption therefore results in a reduction of inspired oxygen concentration. This is due to the fact that in the event of increased oxygen consumption the oxygen concentration of the expired gas declines. Consequently, increased oxygen consumption with low fresh gas flow and a high share of oxygen-depleted rebreathing volume results in a greater reduction of the inspired oxygen concentration than with high fresh gas flow and correspondingly low share of oxygen-depleted rebreathing volume (Figure 3.5).

3.2   Nitrous oxide

3.2.1   Nitrous oxide uptake

The uptake of nitrous oxide follows an exponential curve: although the nitrous oxide uptake decreases rapidly, it is necessary initially to feed great volumes of nitrous oxide into the breathing system. After this initial period of anaesthesia, lasting about 20–30 min, the further decrease in uptake proceeds very slowly, so that nitrous oxide uptake is virtually constant over lengthy periods. According to Severinghaus[16], and assuming an inspired nitrous oxide concentration of about 80% ($FiN_2O = 0.8$), the nitrous oxide uptake of a normal-weight adult can be approximated by means of the following formula:

$$\dot{V}N_2O = 1000 \times t^{-1/2}\,(ml/min)$$

where $t =$ time (min).

This nitrous oxide uptake characteristic, which corresponds to an exponential function, has been confirmed by Barton and Nunn[17], Spieß[18] and Westenskow et al.[7,8] in the range calculated in accordance with the Severinghaus formula.

For calculation of nitrous oxide uptake during the time course of anaesthesia assuming an inspired nitrous oxide concentration of 75% by vol., Beatty[19] quotes the following formula:

$$\dot{V}N_2O = 412 \times t^{-0.37}\,(ml/min)$$

The values calculated with this formula are somewhat lower than those calculated using the Severinghaus formula. A significant correlation with body weight or age of the patients could not be established by Beatty[19].

3.2.2   Implications for anaesthetic practice

An inspired nitrous oxide concentration of 60–65% permits a satisfactory utilization of the nitrous oxide effect, since the state of amnalgesia with adequate somnolence and distinct analgesia can be attained with this concentration[20]. At the same time, this value corresponds to the recommended inspired oxygen concentration of 30% ($FiO_2 = 0.3$). The potential to vary these two values, however, is rather limited for safety reasons[17]. A desired oxygen–nitrous oxide mixture can easily be attained using a high fresh gas flow since, with increasing flow, the composition of fresh gas and inspired gas are almost identical. In the case of low fresh gas flows, consideration must be given to the following problem: the oxygen uptake is constant within certain limits, while the nitrous oxide uptake decreases continuously, corresponding to an exponential function (Figure 3.6).

Should the fresh gas flow be reduced very early, the volume of nitrous oxide extracted from the system is considerably greater than the volume of oxygen taken up by the patient. The FiN_2O drops while the FiO_2 rises. And

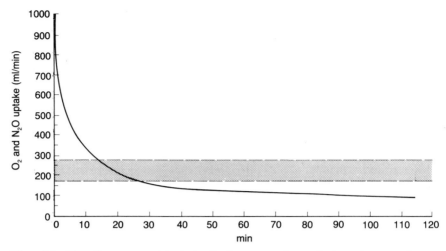

Figure 3.6 While the oxygen uptake during the time course of anaesthesia can be assumed as being constant within certain limits (hatched area), the nitrous oxide uptake decreases exponentially (uptake calculated for a normal-weight adult patient)

if, during the initial phase of anaesthesia, the nitrous oxide volume fed into the system with the fresh gas is even lower than the nitrous oxide uptake, this may result in a gas volume deficiency. On the other hand, in the case of long-term anaesthesia, the nitrous oxide uptake drops to comparatively low values. If now the nitrous oxide volume fed into the system becomes greater than the nitrous oxide uptake, in low flow anaesthesia nitrous oxide is liable to accumulate in the system. Correspondingly the FiN_2O increases, and the FiO_2 decreases.

This is why Lin and Mostert[21] recommend that a 'wash-in phase' with high fresh gas flow should precede the flow reduction. Thereafter, the nitrous oxide uptake remains virtually constant over a long period of time so that a nitrous oxide flow $\dot{V}_fN_2O$ calculated in accordance with the following formula:

$$\dot{V}_fN_2O = 200 \times \text{desired } FiN_2O \text{ (ml/min)}$$

and an oxygen flow being equal to the oxygen uptake delivered as the total fresh gas flow will suffice to ensure the desired composition of inspired gas.

Smith[22], however, comes to the conclusion that, in the individual case, it will not be possible to make an adequately precise calculation for the composition of inspired gas with any one of these different formulae. The lower the fresh gas flow, the greater are the deviations between calculated and measured concentrations. Given a flow of less than 0.9 l/min, no correlation can be established between the oxygen and nitrous oxide concentrations of the fresh gas and that of the anaesthetic gas.

This makes continuous monitoring of the inspired oxygen concentration an inevitable requirement to guarantee an adequate oxygen supply and thus the patient's safety, if anaesthesia is performed with reduced fresh gas flows using a nitrous oxide–oxygen mixture.

3.3   Volatile anaesthetics

3.3.1   Uptake of volatile anaesthetics

3.3.1.1   *Pharmacokinetics of volatile anaesthetics*

Volatile anaesthetics are administered with the objective of attaining an anaesthetic concentration in the central nervous system which affords an adequate pain relief in surgical interventions, and sufficient reduction of consciousness and reflexes at the same time. The amount of anaesthetic required for this purpose must be supplied to the patient's lungs via the breathing system. There the anaesthetic gas or vapour is absorbed by the blood and transported to all organs and tissues, including the brain. The amount of anaesthetic agent entering this tissue compartment brings about anaesthesia. Following a certain period of saturation, it attains the concentration required for sufficient supression of central nervous tissue functions. Bearing this process in mind, it can clearly be recognized that the uptake of volatile anaesthetics is influenced by a great number of physiological, physicochemical and technical factors.

The transport to the lungs is effected via the whole gas-carrying system which consists of the alveolar space, the conducting airways, the breathing system, and possibly a ventilator. The kinetic parameters which influence the uptake in this system are:

- the alveolar minute ventilation volume $\dot{V}_A$ and
- the anaesthetic alveolar concentration C_A.

Transition into the blood is effected via the alveolar membrane. This stage of the mechanism of anaesthetic uptake is determined by:

- the alveolar–capillary concentration difference and
- the blood/gas partition coefficient of the anaesthetic selected $\lambda_{B/G}$.

The blood serves as the carrier for the anaesthetic agent. This convective transport is a function of:

- the cardiac output $\dot{Q}$ and
- the anaesthetic arterial concentration C_a.

The transition into the particular tissue compartment, the diffusion transport, is the ultimate stage of anaesthetic uptake and is determined by:

- the organ blood flow $\dot{Q}_T$
- the organ's tissue volume V_T
- the blood/tissue partial pressure difference of the anaesthetic agent and
- the tissue and agent specific tissue/blood partition coefficient $\lambda_{T/B}$.

The total uptake is the sum of the uptakes of all organs, whereby the relevant virtual distribution volume of the individual organ is calculated by multiplying the organ's volume by its specific tissue/blood partition coefficient[23].

Since diffusion transport proceeds rapidly, the concentration of the anaesthetic in the venous limb of the organ's vessel system corresponds to the agent's tissue concentration. This means that the velocity of uptake is mainly determined by the velocity of the convective transport. The anaesthetist, however, is only able to exert an influence on the kinetic parameters determining the agent's transport to the lung. He has no direct influence on the factors influencing the convection and diffusion transport. From the pharmacokinetic point of view, closed and low flow systems are nothing but a special parameter selection with respect to the rebreathing fraction in establishing the desired alveolar concentration of the inhalational anaesthetic[24].

In order to achieve a constant alveolar concentration in non-rebreathing systems, consideration must be given to three different subsets which comprise the BET scheme (22):

- the amount of anaesthetic agent saturating the alveolar space with the desired concentration (Bolus)
- the substitution of the amount of agent eliminated with the gas exchange caused by the alveolar ventilation (Elimination)
- the substitution of the total anaesthetic uptake, that is, the sum of the uptakes of all individual organs, which can be calculated with the Zuntz equation (Transfer):

$$\dot{V}_A \times C_i = V_A \times C_A + \dot{V}_A \times C_A + C_A \times \lambda_{B/G} \times \Sigma\dot{Q}_T \times e^{-\frac{\dot{Q}_T \times t}{V_T \times \lambda_{B/G}}}$$

$\dot{V}_A \times C_i$ volume of anaesthetic vapour which has to be supplied per unit time (inspiratory supply)

$V_A \times C_A$ saturation of the alveolar space (bolus)

$\dot{V}_A \times C_A$ substitution of the anaesthetic volume being eliminated by alveolar ventilation (elimination)

$$C_A \times \lambda_{B/G} \times \Sigma\dot{Q}_T \times e^{-\frac{\dot{Q}_T \times t}{V_T \times \lambda_{B/G}}}$$

     substitution of the total uptake (transfer)

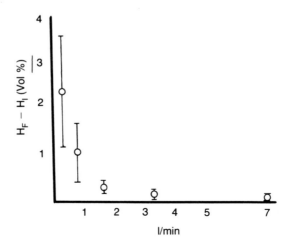

Figure 3.7   The difference between the inspired (H_I) and the fresh gas halothane concentration (H_F) (y-axis) increases with decreasing fresh gas flow (x-axis) (From Baer[27], by permission)

Pharmacokinetic formulae of this complexity, however, do not provide practical assistance in the dosage of volatile anaesthetics, unless a computer and appropriate software is available at the workplace[25,26].

Since the difference between the anaesthetic concentration of the fresh gas and that of the inspired gas increases with progressive reduction of the fresh gas flow (Figure 3.7) and since a relationship between both figures can no longer be established if the fresh gas flow is less than about 1.5 l/min[17], dosage aids must be provided. This is of particular importance if no monitoring is available for measuring the concentration of volatile anaesthetics within the breathing system.

A poll prompted by Tammisto[28] revealed that even experienced anaesthetists could not estimate the inspired anaesthetic concentration in a rebreathing system precisely, although the fresh gas flow and vaporizer settings were known.

3.3.1.2   The Lowe uptake model

Based on the Severinghaus nitrous oxide uptake formula[16], Lowe[6,29] worked out a mathematical concept which approximates the uptake of volatile anaesthetics as a function of the square root of time:

$$\dot{V}_{AN} = C_a \times \dot{Q} \times t^{-1/2} \tag{1}$$

where $\dot{Q}$ = cardiac output (dl/min)
C_a = arterial concentration
t = time (min).

Calculation of the arterial anaesthetic concentration:

$$C_a = C_A \times \lambda_{B/G} \tag{2}$$

where C_A = alveolar concentration
$\lambda_{B/G}$ = blood/gas partition coefficient.

Calculation of the anaesthetic alveolar concentration as a multiple of MAC:

$$C_A = f \times MAC \tag{3}$$

where f = calculating factor, which defines the aspired alveolar concentration as a fraction of MAC
MAC = minimum alveolar concentration.

Calculation of the factor f for the AD_{95} concentration (inhalational anaesthetic concentration ensuring sufficient anaesthetic depth for skin incision in 95% of all patients):

$$f = 1.3 - FiN_2O \tag{4}$$

where FiN_2O = inspired nitrous oxide fraction.

Calculation of the cardiac output according to the Brody formula:

$$\dot{Q} = 2 \times BW(kg)^{3/4} \tag{5}$$

where $BW(kg)$ = patient's body weight in kilograms.

Substitute eqns (2)–(5) in (1):

$$\dot{V}_{AN} = (1.3 - FiN_2O) \times MAC \times \lambda_{B/G} \times 2 \times BW(kg)^{3/4} \times t^{-1/2} \tag{6}$$

By integration of this equation the cumulative dose can be calculated (i.e. the total amount of anaesthetic agent delivered to the patient during the time t):

$$K_D = 2 \times (1.3 - FiN_2O) \times MAC \times \lambda_{B/G} \times 2 \times BW(kg)^{3/4} \times \sqrt{t} + c \tag{7}$$

where c = arterial prime dose.

At the beginning of anaesthesia, a priming dose (P_D) must be fed into the system by means of which the desired concentration of the anaesthetic can be established in the whole gas-carrying space (volume of the lungs, the breathing system, and the ventilator), as well as in the blood:

$$P_D = C_A \times (V_S + V_L) + C_a \times \dot{Q} \tag{8}$$

where $C_A \times (V_S + V_L)$ = prime dose for the gas-carrying compartments
$\qquad C_a \times \dot{Q}$ = prime dose for the blood ($=c$: arterial prime dose)
$\qquad V_S$ = volume of the breathing system (dl)
$\qquad V_L$ = gas volume of the lungs and the airways (dl).

Substitute (2) and (3) in (8):

$$P_D = f \times MAC \times (V_S + V_L) + f \times MAC \times \lambda_{B/G} \times \dot{Q} \tag{9}$$

If the sum of V_S and V_L is assumed to be about 10 litres ($= 100\,dl$), the resultant prime dose can be calculated as follows:

$$P_D = f \times MAC \times (100 + \lambda_{B/G} \times \dot{Q}) \tag{10}$$

Lowe called the dose to be administered after the first minute the unit dose (U_D):

$$U_D = 2 \times C_a \times \dot{Q} \text{ (ml anaesthetic vapour)}$$

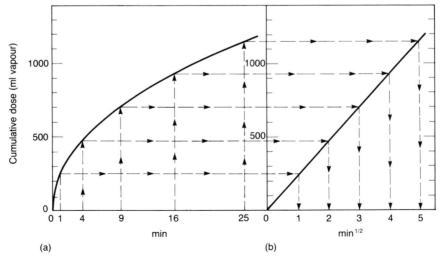

Figure 3.8 Cumulative halothane dose for a patient of 100 kg body weight: in diagram (a) plotted against time t, in diagram (b) against $\sqrt{t}$. The volumes of halothane vapour uptake are identical during whole-numbered $\sqrt{t}$ intervals (From Lowe et al.[6], by permission)

and recommended, the administration of this unit dose in continuously increasing time intervals, that is, after the 1st, 4th, 9th, 16th, etc., minutes. At all these times, the cumulative dose required for maintaining anaesthesia is always a whole-numbered multiple of the unit dose. This results in a dosage scheme for closed system anaesthesia with volatile anaesthetics in which a constant dose of the anaesthetic agent is administered at each time at which $\sqrt{t}$ becomes a whole-numbered figure (Figure 3.8b).

3.3.1.3   The Westenskow uptake model

Westenskow et al.[30], Thomson et al.[31] and Gorsky et al.[32] pointed out, however, that the doses of inhalational anaesthetic agents calculated according to Lowe's uptake model are too high and that the anaesthetic concentrations are about 25–50% above the desired values (Figure 3.9).

Westenskow summarizes the results of his investigations concerning uptake as follows: The uptake of volatile anaesthetics is neither constant nor does it follow the 'square-root of time' rule of the Lowe model. With semi-logarithmic presentation, the anaesthetic uptake can be described by two straight lines whose intersection point divides anaesthesia into two phases: during the first 10 minutes, the uptake is high and decreases rapidly, while in the second phase the uptake remains almost constant (Figure 3.10).

This graph results from the calculation of average values of enflurane uptake obtained from 23 patients. Westenskow et al.[30] and Zbinden[33] stress,

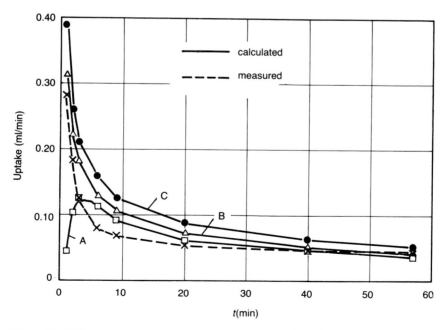

Figure 3.9   Difference in halothane uptake between measured values (---) and figures calculated according to the Lowe formula (——) (From Thomson et al.[31], by permission)

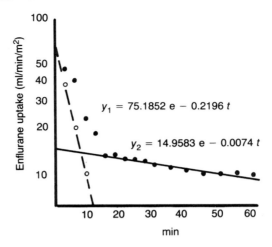

Figure 3.10   In semi-logarithmic presentation, the enflurane uptake during the time course of anaesthesia can be plotted by means of two straight regression lines. The intersection (after 10 min) splits anaesthesia into two phases with different uptake characteristics: the vessel-rich tissues are saturated during the first phase and poorly vascularized tissues in the second phase (From Westenskow et al.[30], by permission)

however, that the uptake may differ greatly in individual cases so that at best the graph can be an orientation aid, but in no way provides more than a guideline on dosage.

3.3.1.4   The Lin uptake model

Following mass spectrometric measurements of the uptake of volatile anaesthetics Lin et al.[21,34] came to the conclusion that the rapid initial rise of the quotient F_A/F_I (end-expired (alveolar) to inspired concentration) is based on the wash-in phase. Depending on the fresh gas flow, this takes about 3–20 min: during that time the gas concentration is established and brought to equilibrium within the whole gas-carrying space. The uptake itself, however, can be assumed to be comparatively constant and is essentially a function of the alveolar–capillary partial pressure difference, provided that the cardiac output and ventilation remain unchanged.

Following equilibrium, the uptake of volatile anaesthetics can be approximated for the following period of about 120 min by using the formulae:

$Uptake_{hal} = 15$–20 ml halothane vapour per % desired concentration

$Uptake_{enf} = 30$ ml enflurane vapour per % desired concentration

In addition, the long time constant of the closed system tends to ensure a constant gas concentration.

Mostert et al.[35] also recommended proceeding as follows: The system should only be closed after an initial phase of anaesthesia with a high fresh gas flow, during which a steady state of gas concentration can be attained.

After flow reduction, the loss of volatile anaesthetic resulting from uptake can be replenished by only small amounts of anaesthetic vapour.

3.3.2   Implications for anaesthetic practice

Based on the aforementioned considerations, the following rules may be derived for clinical practice:

1. There is no generally accepted dosage pattern for a change from the habitual anaesthetic method with semi-closed system in which gas concentrations are stabilized in flowing steady state, to the quantitative system of equilibrium using a closed breathing system.
2. Each dosage pattern and every pharmacokinetic calculation model will merely offer an aid to orientation. When used in anaesthetic practice, it requires critical verification by careful observation of the individual patient and may have to be adjusted during the course of anaesthesia. This rule is, though, also applicable to anaesthesia management with a high fresh gas flow.
3. It should not be overlooked that the goal of such dosage patterns is to establish desired values for anaesthetic concentrations. No statement can be made as to whether in the individual case the resultant depth of anaesthesia attained with this concentration is adequate for the respective surgical intervention or the individual reaction of the patient.

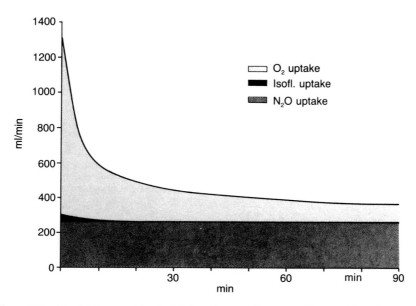

Figure 3.11   The total gas uptake depicted as the sum of oxygen, nitrous oxide and anaesthetic vapour uptake. Calculated for a patient of 75 kg body weight, an inspired nitrous oxide concentration of 65% by volume, and an expiratory isoflurane concentration of 0.75% by volume

4. The initial phase of anaesthesia is marked by a great demand for nitrous oxide and volatile anaesthetic. In practice, it is of minor significance whether this can be explained by the wash-in process into the gas-carrying space itself or by the high uptake during the induction phase. But at the time when the fresh gas flow is reduced, it must be critically examined whether the selected flow covers the current demand for nitrous oxide and anaesthetic vapour. Otherwise, undesired changes in anaesthetic depth and deficiency of gas volume in the system may result.

3.4   Total gas uptake

The total gas uptake is calculated from the sum of oxygen, nitrous oxide and anaesthetic vapour volumes being taken up at the particular time during anaesthesia. The uptake of nitrous oxide and volatile anaesthetics follows an exponential function, while the uptake of oxygen can be assumed as being constant within certain limits. To this end, the total gas uptake thus decreases with time during the course of anaesthesia (Figure 3.11).

3.5   References

1. Brody, S. *Bioenergetics and Growth*, Reinhold, New York (1945)
2. Kleiber, M. Body size and metabolic rate. *Physiol. Rev.*, **27**, 511–539 (1949)
3. Arndt, G. and Stock, M. Ch. Brody's equation: a reinterpretation and its clinical application. *Circular*, **5**, 5–8 (1988)
4. Arndt, J. O. Inhalationsanästhetika und Stoffwechsel: O_2-Verbrauch wacher, schlafender oder narkotisierter Hunde unter Grundumsatzbedingungen. In *Die Inhaltionsnarkose: Steuerung und Überwachung* (eds H. Schwilden and H. Stoeckel), INA-Schriftenreihe, Bol. 58, Thieme, Stuttgart (1987), pp. 43–52
5. Guyton, A. C., Jones, C. E. and Coleman, T. C. *Circulatory Physiology: Cardiac Output and its Regulations*, Saunders, Philadelphia (1973), pp. 12–14 and 21–24
6. Lowe, H. J. and E. A. Ernst, E. A. *The Quantitative Practice of Anesthesia*, Williams and Wilkins, Baltimore (1981)
7. Westenskow, D. R., Jordan, W. S. and Gehmlich, D. S. Electronic feedback control and measurement of oxygen consumption during closed circuit anaesthesia. In *Low Flow and Closed System Anesthesia* (eds J. A. Aldrete, H. J. Lowe and R. W. Virtue), Grune and Stratton, New York (1979), pp. 135–146
8. Westenskow, D. R. and Jordan, W. S. Automatic control of closed circuit anesthesia and the measurement of Enflurane, N_2O and oxygen uptake. In *Geschlossenes System für Inhalationsnarkosen*, Internationales Symposium, Düsseldorf, 7–8 May 1982 (Abstract)
9. Manawadu, B. R., Hartwig, F. E., Sherrill, D. and Swanson, G. D. Monitoring oxygen consumption utilizing low flow techniques. In *Low Flow and Closed System Anesthesia* (eds J. A. Aldrete, H. J. Lowe and R. W. Virtue), Grune and Stratton, New York (1979), pp. 147–150
10. Finsterer, U. Lungenfunktion unter Narkose. *Anästh. Intensivmed.* **24**, 277–287 (1983)
11. Reineke, H. Respiratorische Risikofaktoren und Narkosebeatmung. *Anästh. Intensivmed.*, **24**, 33–36 (1983)
12. Don, H. Hypoxemia and hypercapnia during and after anesthesia. In *Complications in Anesthesiology* (eds F. K. Orkin and L. H. Cooperman), Lippincott, Philadelphia (1983), pp. 183–207
13. Schilling, R. and Weis, K. H. Zur Sauerstoffkonzentration im Narkosesystem. *Anaesthesist*, **22**, 198–201 (1973)

14. Schreiber, P. Anesthesia systems. In *North American Draeger Safety Guidelines*, Merchants Press, Boston (1985)
15. Westenskow, D. R. How much oxygen? *Int. J. Clin. Monitor. Comput.*, **2**, 187–189 (1986)
16. Severinghaus, J. W. The rate of uptake of nitrous oxide in man. *J. Clin. Invest.*, **33**, 1183–1189 (1954)
17. Barton, F. and Nunn, J. F. Totally closed circuit nitrous oxide/oxygen anaesthesia. *Br. J. Anaesth.*, **47**, 350–357 (1975)
18. Spieß, W. Narkose im geschlossenen System mit kontinuierlicher inspiratorischer Sauerstoffmessung. *Anaesthesist*, **26**, 503–513 (1977)
19. Beatty, P. C. W., Kay, B. and Healy, T. E. J. Measurement of the rates of nitrous oxide uptake and nitrogen excretion in man. *Br. J. Anaesth.*, **56**, 232–232 (1984)
20. Parbrook, G. D. The levels of nitrous oxide analgesia. *Br. J. Anaesth.*, **39**, 974–982 (1967)
21. Lin, C. Y. and Mostert, J. W. Inspired O_2 and N_2O concentrations in essentially closed circuits. *Anaesthesist*, **26**, 514–517 (1977)
22. Smith, T. C. Nitrous oxide and low flow inflow circle systems. *Anesthesiology*, **27**, 266–271 (1966)
23. Schwilden, H., Stoeckel, H., Lauven, P. M. and Schüttler, J. Pharmakokinetik und MAC – Praktische Implikationen für die Dosierung volatiler Anästhetika. In *Inhalationsanästhetika. Anästhesiologie und Intensivmedizin* (eds K. Peter, B. R. Brown, E. Martin and O. Norlander), Bd. 184, Springer, Berlin (1986), pp. 18–26
24. Schwilden, H., Stoeckel, H., Lauven P. M. and Schüttler, J. Pharmakokinetik der Inhalationsanästhetika. In *Geschlossenes System für Inhalationsnarkosen*, Internationales Symposium, Düsseldorf, 7–8 May 1982 (Abstract)
25. Schwilden, H. *Narkosesimulator*, Deutsche Abbott, Wiesbaden (1986)
26. Schwilden, H. Die rechnergestützte interaktive Dosierung volatiler Anästhetika (AC-Prädiktor). In *Die Inhalationsnarkose: Steuerung und Überwachung* (eds H. Schwilden and H. Stoeckel), INA Bd. 58, Thieme, Stuttgart (1987), pp. 167–173
27. Baer, B. Die Abhängigkeit der inspiratorischen Halothankonzentration im Kreisystem von der Höhe der Frischgaszufuhr. *Anaesthesist*, **32**, 6–11 (1983)
28. Tammisto, T. Monitoring der Konzentration volatiler Anästhetika. In *Die Inhalationsnarkose: Steuerung und Überwachung* (eds H. Schwilden and H. Stoeckel), INA Bd. 58, Thieme, Stuttgart (1987), pp. 33–38
29. Lowe, H. J. *Dose-Regulated Penthrane Anesthesia*, Abbott Laboratories, Chicago (1972)
30. Westenskow, D. R., Jordan, W. S. and Hayes, J. K. Uptake of enflurane: a study of the variability between patients. *Br. J. Anaesth.*, **55**, 598–610 (1983)
31. Thomson, D., Zbinden, A. and Westenskow, D. Pharmakokinetik von Inhalationsanästhetika – Untersuchungen mit einem feed-back kontrollierten geschlossenen System. In *Inhalationsanästhetika. Anästhesiologie und Intensivmedizin* (eds K. Peter, B. R. Brown, E. Martin and O. Norlander), Bd. 184, Springer, Berlin (1986), pp. 34–42
32. Gorsky, B. H., Hall, R. L. and Redford, J. E. A compromise for closed system anesthesia. *Anesth. Analg.*, **57**, 18–24 (1978)
33. Zbinden, A. M. *Inhalationsanästhetika: Aufnahme und Verteilung*, Wissenschaftliche Verlagsabteilung, Deutsche Abbott, Wiesbaden (1987)
34. Lin, C. Y., Mostert, J. W. and Benson, D. W. Closed circle systems. A new direction in the practice of anaesthesia. *Acta Anaesth. Scand.*, **24**, 354–361 (1980)
35. Mostert, J. W., Goldberg, I. S., Lanzl, E. F. and Lowe, H. J. Das geschlossene System. *Anaesthesist*, **26**, 495–502 (1977)

4

Anaesthetic methods with reduced fresh gas flow

Depending on the selection of the fresh gas flow, rebreathing systems may be semi-open, semi-closed or closed. The rebreathing volume increases as the fresh gas flow declines, while simultaneouslythe excess gas volume decreases. With semi-closed use of a rebreathing system, the fresh gas fed into the system can be arbitrarily set to any value that is less than the minute volume, but greater than the total gas uptake of the patient. However, the fresh gas flow must at least equal that volume, which is taken up by the patient at any given time or is lost through leaks. Only by supplying at least this amount of gas will the appropriate gas volume for ventilation be available.

Contrary to White[1] the author suggests that the term 'low flow' should not be linked to a defined fresh gas flow rate, but rather to the proportion of rebreathing. 'Low flow' will thus be defined as a fresh gas flow so low as to raise the rebreathing fraction to at least 50% of the exhaled gas volume. This definition seems to be the more justifiable, as the share of rebreathing not only depends on the fresh gas flow, but also on the fresh gas utilization of the respective breathing system and the patient's individual total gas uptake. If, for instance, a breathing system is used which makes inefficient use of fresh gas, a comparatively high flow would then be already sufficient to realize low flow anaesthesia; whereas in paediatric anaesthesia, using a system featuring excellent fresh gas utilization, low flow anaesthesia would only require a minimal flow rate.

If the proportion of rebreathing is depicted by the percentage of exhaled carbon dioxide (Figure 4.1) actually reaching the absorber, the following can be demonstrated. Using modern rebreathing circle absorber systems featuring sufficiently good fresh gas utilization on adult patients, the proportion of rebreathing will only exceed 50% if the flow is reduced to less than 2 l/min. Thus, in the following discussion on low flow anaesthesia only those anaesthetic techniques which are performed with fresh gas flows in this range will be taken into consideration.

A number of different variants of anaesthesia management with low fresh gas flow are described in the literature (Figure 4.2). All the different techniques have in common a more or less lengthy initial phase, during which a high fresh gas flow is used to flush the anaesthetic gas into the system. Simultaneously, nitrogen is washed out of the system. In the case of closed system anaesthesia, the fresh gas flow is reduced to just that volume taken up by the patient or lost via leakages. Since the total gas uptake lessens gradually during anaesthesia, the fresh gas flow must be continuously adapted to the changing uptake. However, if one succeeds in adapting not only the volume of the fresh gas, but also its composition to the current oxygen, nitrous oxide and volatile agent uptake, this will be the realization of quantitative closed system anaesthesia. The gas composition within the

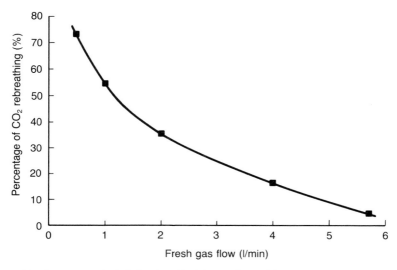

Figure 4.1   Percentage of exhaled carbon dioxide actually reaching the absorber as a function of the fresh gas flow. Measurements at a circle absorption system 8 ISO (Drägerwerk, Lübeck), Pat. R.S.: 72 kg, 182 cm, ventilatory minute volume 5.7 l/min

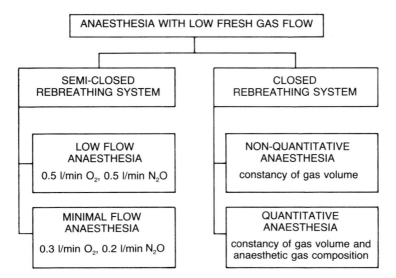

Figure 4.2   Different techniques of anaesthesia management with low fresh gas flows

breathing system would then remain constant during the whole time course of anaesthesia.

There are, however, alternative methods to closed system anaesthesia. For reasons of practicability, and although rebreathing is used extensively, they are characterized by the use of a small excess of fresh gas. Minimal flow anaesthesia is performed with a fresh gas flow of 0.5 l/min[2,3] and low flow anaesthesia with a fresh gas flow of 1.0 l/min[4,5]. Both anaesthetic methods can thus be considered as extreme variants of semi-closed anaesthetic management.

All the different techniques of anaesthesia management with low fresh gas flow (Table 4.1) have in common that, over the time course of anaesthesia, the fresh gas flow is more or less precisely adapted to the total gas uptake (Figure 4.3). This is the basic principle of reducing excess gas volumes discharged from the system, and of using the advantages of rebreathing to their utmost extent.

Table 4.1   Anaesthetic techniques using low fresh gas flows

LOW FLOW ANAESTHESIA[4]

Fresh gas flow	constant 1.0 l/min
Fresh gas composition	50% O_2, 50% N_2O
Rebreathing	partial
Use of excess gas	yes
Anaesthetic gas composition	changes with the course of anaesthesia
Technical classification	semi-closed rebreathing system

MINIMAL FLOW ANAESTHESIA[2]

Fresh gas flow	constant 0.5 l/min
Fresh gas composition	60% O_2, 40% N_2O
Rebreathing	extensive
Use of excess gas	minimal
Anaesthetic gas composition	changes with the course of anaesthesia
Technical classification	semi-closed rebreathing system

NON-QUANTITATIVE CLOSED SYSTEM ANAESTHESIA[26]

Fresh gas flow	intermittent adaptation of fresh gas volume to gas loss via uptake or leakages
Fresh gas composition	varies, intermittent alteration of the anaesthetic gas composition
Rebreathing	entire exhaled gas after carbon dioxide elimination
Use of excess gas	no
Anaesthetic gas composition	varies during the course of anaesthesia
Technical classification	closed rebreathing system

QUANTITATIVE CLOSED SYSTEM ANAESTHESIA[20]

Fresh gas flow	continuous adaptation of fresh gas flow to the individual total gas uptake
Fresh gas composition	varies, continuous adaptation to individual uptake of anaesthetic gas components
Rebreathing	entire exhaled gas after carbon dioxide elimination
Use of excess gas	no
Anaesthetic gas composition	constant during the whole course of anaesthesia according to preset values
Technical classification	closed rebreathing system

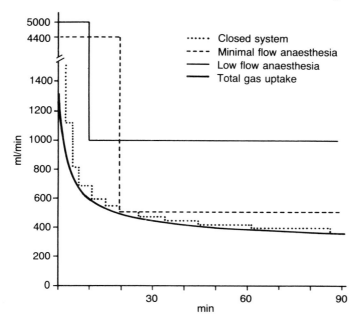

Figure 4.3   Common characteristics of anaesthetic techniques with low fresh gas flow. Following an initial phase using high gas flow, the fresh gas flow rate is reduced and thus adapted to the total gas uptake which continuously decreases during the course of anaesthesia. To achieve the most precise adaptation, frequent adjustments of the flowmeters are required.

4.1   Low flow anaesthesia

This anaesthetic technique, in which the fresh gas flow is reduced to 1 l/min, was published by Foldes and co-workers in 1952. As Sir Francis related, none of the anaesthesia journals would accept his paper, so that it had to be published in the *Annals of Surgery*[4]. After having used this technique in more than 10 000 cases, the results were summarized as follows:

The oxygen concentration in the breathing system decreases

- if, with constant fresh gas composition, the fresh gas flow is reduced
- if, with constant flow, the fresh gas composition is changed in favour of nitrous oxide, and
- if, with unchanged fresh gas composition and constant flow, the duration of the anaesthesia increases.

For calculation of the oxygen and nitrous oxide flows by means of which a desired oxygen concentration can be attained in the system at a preselected fresh gas flow, Foldes quoted a simple formula:

$$\dot{V}_f O_2 = \dot{V}O_2 + ((\dot{V}_f - \dot{V}O_2)/100) \times FiO_2$$

$$\dot{V}_f N_2O = \dot{V}_f - \dot{V}_f O_2$$

where $\dot{V}_fO_2$ = oxygen flow required
       $\dot{V}_fN_2O$ = nitrous oxide flow required
       $\dot{V}_f$ = fresh gas flow
       $\dot{V}O_2$ = calculated oxygen consumption
       FiO_2 = desired inspired oxygen fraction

Foldes and colleagues suggested the following procedure for performance of low flow anaesthesia:

(a) Initial selection of a high fresh gas flow for 3 minutes (4 l/min N_2O, 1–1.5 l/min O_2).
(b) Thereafter, reduction of the fresh gas flow to 1 l/min, whereby the respective oxygen and nitrous oxide flow should equal the gas volumes calculated from the formula.
(c) Should the breathing system be opened to atmosphere for some reason, steps (a) and (b) have to be repeated.
(d) Where patients with a high metabolic rate are concerned, a correspondingly higher inspired oxygen concentration must be given.

With a standardized setting of the fresh gas composition (0.5 l/min O_2, 0.5 l/min N_2O), an average inspired oxygen concentration of $30 \pm 5\%$ was attained, and in no case did this value drop below 20%.

In 1985, Foldes and Duncalf presented a somewhat modified concept[5]. The flow reduction is preceded by an initial phase lasting 10 min with high fresh gas flow (2 l/min O_2, 3 l/min N_2O), to ensure adequate denitrogenation. Thereafter, a standard fresh gas flow of 1 l/min (0.5 l/min O_2, 0.5 l/min N_2O) should be set. Since nitrous oxide uptake decreases continuously during the course of anaesthesia, Foldes recommended modifying the fresh gas composition after another 10 min to 0.7 l/min O_2 and 0.3 l/min N_2O. Should rapid changes in concentrations be necessary, the fresh gas flow should be increased.

Foldes prefers low flow anaesthesia to methods with an even lower fresh gas volume, proposing the following arguments:

- the technique of low flow anaesthesia can easily be learned
- the monitoring demands, oxygen and carbon dioxide measurement, as specified by Foldes, are low
- the demands placed on gas tightness of the system can easily be satisfied with routine maintenance of the machines
- the dosage of volatile anaesthetics is easy and simple
- with a flow lower than 1 l/min, even minor inaccuracies of the flow control of oxygen and nitrous oxide may result in grave alterations of oxygen concentration within the breathing system
- with an even lower flow, special water traps will be required
- the advantages of a further fresh gas flow reduction, and thus further improved utilization of rebreathing, are rather insignificant, whereas anaesthesia management will become considerably more difficult.

The low flow technique was somewhat modified by Grote et al.[6]: following an initial phase with high flow (2 l/min O_2, 4 l/min N_2O) over 5 min, they also recommend fresh gas flow reduction to 1 l/min (0.5 l/min O_2, 0.5 l/min N_2O). According to Grote, the inspiratory oxygen concentration never drops below 30% with these standardized settings, so that they even considered continuous oxygen measurement unnecessary. However, they recommended changing the fresh gas composition after 1–2 h to 0.6 l/min O_2 and 0.4 l/min N_2O.

Grote and colleagues also judge low flow anaesthesia as being advantageous since it is easily understood and simple in performance. However, they emphasize that closed system anaesthesia should be preferred if adequate monitoring devices are available for measuring the concentrations of oxygen and volatile anaesthetics in the gas mixture.

4.2   Minimal flow anaesthesia

In 1974, Virtue[2] introduced an anaesthetic method, termed 'minimal flow anaesthesia', in which the fresh gas flow is reduced to 0.5 l/min. This method could be performed without risk of hypoxia, since in those days, devices for continuous monitoring of the inspiratory oxygen concentration were already available.

Following induction in the usual manner, relaxation, intubation and controlled ventilation, anaesthesia is initially performed with a high fresh gas flow (1.5 l/min O_2, 3.5 l/min N_2O) for 15–20 min. During this phase, nitrogen is washed out of the body and the breathing system. Adequate volumes of nitrous oxide and anaesthetic vapour corresponding to the initially high uptake are fed into the system so that the desired concentrations can be established and homogenized in the entire gas-carrying space. After this initial phase using high flow, the fresh gas volume is reduced to a standardized setting of 0.5 l/min and simultaneously its composition changed to 60% O_2 (0.3 l/min O_2) and 40% N_2O (0.2 l/min N_2O). For a patient of 80-kg body weight, the oxygen consumption can be calculated according to the Brody formula (see Section 3.1.1), at 267 ml/min, and the nitrous oxide uptake is calculated after 20 min according to the Severinghaus formula (see Section 3.2.1), at 223 ml/min. Thus, after flow reduction, oxygen is administered in excess, while the nitrous oxide fed into the system is somewhat less than the actual uptake. It must be considered, though, that the nitrous oxide uptake decreases exponentially, so that after another 10 min it amounts to only 183 ml/min for the given patient. That in turn means that, at this time, nitrous oxide is also being fed into the breathing system in excess. With patients of lower weight, the excess gas volume is accordingly higher. Thus, minimal flow anaesthesia is an extreme variant of semi-closed system anaesthesia, using the lowest practicable excess gas volume and virtually complete rebreathing.

It goes without saying that, with such low fresh gas volumes of standardized composition, the question of the course of the inspiratory oxygen concentration had to be answered by Virtue. On average, the FiO_2 drops within a period of 120 min, from an initial value of 0.42 to 0.33, and after an anaesthetic duration of 3 h to a value of 0.29. The lowest value measured in an individual case was 0.22 after 3 h[2]. The decrease in the inspired oxygen concentration depending on the duration of the anaesthetic procedure can be attributed to the fact, that with increasingly low nitrous oxide uptake this gas accumulates in the breathing system. This is why Virtue recommends that, where patients of more than 80-kg body weight are concerned, the inspiratory oxygen concentration should be monitored continuously. Whenever the oxygen concentration drops to the lower limit, the oxygen flow should be increased. Alternatively, a higher fresh gas flow with higher oxygen portion, about 400 ml/min O_2, 200 ml/min N_2O, could be used right from the beginning. Compared with low flow anaesthesia, there is no essential difference with respect to the inspiratory oxygen concentration: within 3 h the FiO_2 drops from initially 0.37 to 0.30.

Vitrue summarizes that an adequate oxygen supply can be ensured over a period of almost 3 h with the recommended fresh gas composition and the use of a 500 ml/min flow.

According to Virtue, the advantages of minimal flow anaesthesia can be attributed to

- an extensive utilization of the advantages inherent in rebreathing
- bridging the initial phase of anaesthesia, during which the patient takes up great volumes of nitrous oxide and anaesthetic vapour, by the use of a high fresh gas flow; during this initial phase, furthermore, nitrogen is washed out completely and the desired gas concentrations are evenly flushed into the system
- the fact that, although the fresh gas flow is considerably reduced, there remains an excess gas volume, which can compensate for leakage losses.

Spieß[7-9] has continuously emphasized the exceptional practicability of this anaesthetic method in routine practice. The disadvantages with respect to closed system anaesthesia are, according to Spieß, the decrease in FiO_2, resulting from the standardized and fixed setting of the fresh gas composition. Furthermore, this method does not enable the anaesthetist to measure precisely oxygen consumption as well as nitrous oxide and volatile anaesthetic uptake[7]. Minimal flow anaesthesia can be performed all the more readily without serious problems if new and advanced anaesthetic machines are used[10].

4.3   Closed system anaesthesia

If the composition of the fresh gas and its volume are precisely adapted to the patient's individual uptake of nitrous oxide, oxygen and volatile anaesthetic, maximal reduction of fresh gas flow will be achieved. Since the fresh gas volume which is fed into the breathing system corresponds quantitatively to the gas volume extracted from the system, the excess gas discharge valve has to be closed. The entire exhalation volume is rebreathed after carbon dioxide absorption. While low flow and minimal flow anaesthesia are performed at constant fresh gas flows, closed system anaesthesia requires continuous adaptation of the fresh gas volume to match the current uptake. This is problematic, especially during the initial phase of anaesthesia, when the uptake of nitrous oxide and volatile anaesthetic, and to a certain extent even oxygen, is subject to rapid changes. Although the management of anaesthesia may be greatly facilitated by a time-limited use of high fresh gas flows, the objective is an early closing of the system, so that advantages of this anaesthetic method may be exploited.

The problems involved in an early transition to closed system anaesthesia were summarized by Nunn[11] as follows:

1. Denitrogenation must be completed prior to closing the breathing system, since otherwise the nitrogen concentration in the system will increase.
2. During the first minutes, the nitrous oxide flow has to be virtually continuously readjusted in accordance with the rapid initial decrease of its uptake.
3. During the initial phase, while anaesthesia is still light, the oxygen consumption may differ considerably from the calculated basic consumption.
4. If the anaesthetic machines used are equipped with vaporizers featuring limited output[12] which are switched into the fresh gas supply (VOC), with early fresh gas flow reduction it will not be possible to administer the amount of vapour corresponding to the initial high uptake of volatile anaesthetic. Thus, the alveolar anaesthetic concentration cannot be kept at the desired constant level. This can be explained by a brief calculation. Given the maximum setting of a halothane vaporizer (i.e. Vapor, Drägerwerk AG, Lübeck: 4%), only 20 ml of halothane vapour are introduced into the system per minute at a fresh gas flow of 0.5 l/min. In accordance with the Lowe uptake formula, a patient of 100 kg, however, requires 148 ml halothane vapour during the first minute to attain an alveolar concentration of $0.65 \times$ MAC, and 50 ml/min during the following 3 min. Only after 16 min does the uptake decline to about 20 ml/min, thus matching the vaporizer's maximum output at a flow of 0.5 l/min. This means that the vaporizer would have to have a maximum output of 20–30% to cover the high initial demand.

The problems discussed may be solved as follows:

1. Denitrogenation can be achieved prior to induction of anaesthesia, if, for a period of at least 5 min, the patient inhales via a face mask pure oxygen which is fed into the system at a high flow rate.
2. With the objective of feeding an adequate nitrous oxide volume rapidly into the system to meet the initially high nitrous oxide uptake, Barton and Nunn[13] recommended proceeding as follows: After rapid denitrogenation as described above, anaesthesia is induced with barbiturate in the usual manner, and the intubated patient is connected to a breathing system previously filled with pure nitrous oxide. Assuming the volume of the system to be 4 litres and the functional residual capacity of the patient as being 2 litres, after a few ventilation cycles the gas of the two compartments is mixed and the alveolar nitrous oxide concentration amounts to about 65%. Thus, the nitrous oxide flow can be immediately set to 0.25 l/min and the oxygen flow to the calculated oxygen demand.

   Ernst[14] recommends that, following denitrogenation and induction of anaesthesia, a high nitrous oxide flow of 6–9 l/min and an oxygen volume of about 0.25–0.3 l/min, which corresponds to the calculated consumption, should be selected. With hyperventilation, it should be possible to achieve a rapid and homogeneous wash-in of the desired gas concentrations of 65% N_2O and 35% O_2 in the entire system. The nitrous oxide flow should be reduced to 0.6 l/min as soon as the FiO_2 has dropped to a value of 0.35. Further corrections of the composition and the volume of the fresh gas should ensure constancy of the gas volume circulating in the system and the desired inspiratory oxygen concentration.

3. The greatest problem involved in an extremely early reduction of the fresh gas flow, however, is the supply of a sufficient amount of anaesthetic vapour, which meets the initially high uptake.

Weingarten[15] and Lowe and Ernst[16] recommend the injection of liquid volatile anaesthetic directly into the breathing system (Figure 4.4). By separating the anaesthetic agent's dosage from that of the fresh gas, it is possible to feed adequate amounts of volatile anaesthetic into the system, independently of the fresh gas flow.

White[17], however, points out that consideration must be given to possible great fluctuations of anaesthetic concentration with such a technique, and that an even and rapid evaporation of volatile anaesthetic cannot be guaranteed without auxiliary equipment such as vaporizer sieves and circle system blowers. Finally there is the danger of inadvertent intravenous injection of the volatile anaesthetic drawn up in a syringe.

Droh[18] suggests the use of vaporizers with a higher output; however, due to national regulations[12] their use on humans is prohibited, for instance, in Germany. This is the reason why the recommendations for an initial vapour

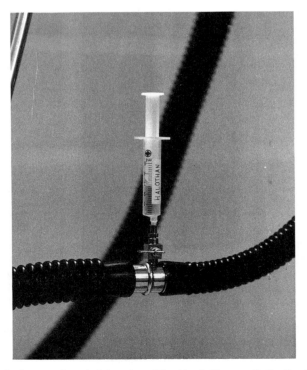

Figure 4.4 Injection port for administration of liquid volatile anaesthetic directly into the expiratory limb of the breathing system

setting (enflurane 7.0%) given by Ernst[14] for the TEC vaporizer cannot be realized.

Another alternative could be the use of vaporizers which are switched into the breathing system (VIC), by means of which the volatile anaesthetic could be administered independently of the fresh gas flow. However, during controlled ventilation the risk of accidental overdose would be so great[17] that this possibility will not be discussed further.

All the different methods mentioned above have been used to try to achieve closed system anaesthesia in spite of grave inadequacies in terms of anaesthetic machinery. The procedure is difficult if conventional anaesthetic machines are used[19]. The control of the volatile agent concentration and the continuous adaptation of fresh gas composition and volume to the nitrous oxide and oxygen uptakes is involved and imprecise, since the technical components for gas dosage are generally not designed for such low gas flows. Frequently, the systems are not sufficiently gas tight and are subject to leaks, while the function of anaesthetic ventilators may also be considerably impaired by the reduction of fresh gas flow.

According to current standards, the following technical requirements must be satisfied to ensure reliable performance of closed system anaesthesia[19,20]:

● high grade gas tightness of the breathing system and the anaesthetic ventilator
● precisely operating low flow control systems for nitrous oxide and oxygen
● precisely operating dosage systems for administration of volatile anaesthetics, featuring an appropriate output and suitable for use with low fresh gas flows
● an anaesthetic ventilator that operates independently of the fresh gas flow
● devices for continuous measurement and monitoring of the anaesthetic gas composition.

These requirements are only satisfied by the new generation of anaesthetic machines. The technical features of these machines are such that they enable the use of closed system anaesthesia.

4.3.1 Non-quantitative closed system anaesthesia

In the author's hospital, closed system anaesthesia was performed with the Cicero anaesthetic workstation (Drägerwerk AG, Lübeck), which features a flowmeter set especially designed for low flow anaesthesia[21]. By means of a computer, the nitrous oxide uptake ($\dot{V}N_2O$) was calculated according to the Severinghaus formula, and the uptake of the anaesthetic selected ($\dot{V}_{an}$) according to the Lowe formula at minute intervals. The oxygen uptake ($\dot{V}O_2$) was calculated by using the Brody formula and assumed to be constant during the course of anaesthesia (see Chapter 3). The respective adjustment of the vaporizer was obtained by calculation of following quotient: $100 \times \dot{V}_{an}/(\dot{V}O_2 + \dot{V}N_2O)$.

After an initial phase lasting between 5 and 15 minutes, during which a high fresh gas flow was applied, the values calculated for the uptake were set at the flowmeter bank and the vaporizer, and were changed at one-minute intervals in accordance with the newly computed values. Possible imbalances in volume between calculated and actual gas uptake were compensated for

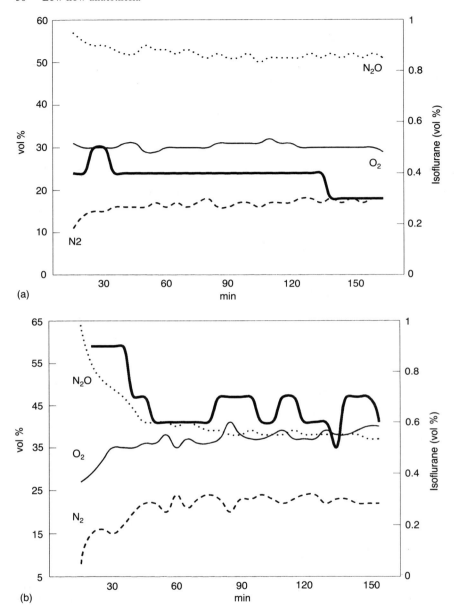

Figure 4.5   Oxygen, nitrous oxide, nitrogen and isuflurane concentrations during the course of two anaesthetics with closed system (Cicero, Drägerwerk, Lübeck). The accumulation of nitrogen results from slow nitrogen washout from the poor vessel group tissues. Also indispensable for performance of closed system anaesthesia, the sampling gas has to be led back into the system after its passage through the gas analyser. Thus, together with the anaesthetic gas, ambient air used as reference or calibration gas may flow into the breathing system and exacerbate nitrogen accumulation. Heavy line: exp. isoflurane concentration. (a) 77-year-old patient, 1.62 m, 66.5 kg nominal value for expired isoflurane concentration 0.5% (b) 49-year-old patient, 1.77 m, 96.5 kg, nominal value for expired isoflurane concentration 0.9%

automatically by the changing filling level of the anaesthetic reservoir bag. If an average filling level of the reservoir was maintained, it could be assumed that the fresh gas flow largely met the total gas uptake. Although in the individual case the measured gas concentrations corresponded well to the chosen set points, and the anaesthetic gas composition did not change considerably during the course of anaesthesia (Figure 4.5a), in most of the cases undertaken with this procedure it was not possible to keep the gas composition as precisely constant as desired (Figure 4.5b). It is obvious that in the individual case there may be considerable differences between the actual and the calculated gas uptake.

Proceeding in the way described, it may be possible to achieve a fresh gas flow reduction down to just that gas volume which is taken up by the patient. This precludes any discharge of excess gas from the system. By definition, the procedure thus corresponds to closed system anaesthesia. However, this technique cannot be defined as being quantitative, since the changes observed in the anaesthetic gas composition can only be explained by an imbalance between the gas volumes fed into the system and the actual nitrous oxide, oxygen and anaesthetic uptake. The term quantitative anaesthesia implies a constancy of composition as well as volume of circulating gas.

In addition, it is evident that in practice it will not be possible for the anaesthetist to change the setting of the vaporizer and the flow control system continually.

4.3.2   Quantitative closed system anaesthesia

Quantitative closed system anaesthesia is practicable only if the dosage of the anaesthetic gases is electronically controlled by closed-loop feedback[21,22]. From the technical point of view this calls for precisely operating gas metering systems[23]. For the first time ever, such a technical concept has been realized in the form of the PhysioFlex machine (Physio, Haarlem, Netherlands)[24]. Oxygen is fed into the system at precisely that volume which will maintain the set inspiratory oxygen concentration. The constancy of the gas volume circulating in the system is guaranteed by an appropriate addition of nitrous oxide and the volatile anaesthetic is injected into the system in liquid form in just such an amount that a preselected expiratory set point is gained within a short time and kept constant at that level. Electronic control of gas metering with closed-loop feedback has proved to be very precise in clinical tests[25]. Provided that the system is absolutely gas tight and gas loss via leakages can be precluded, the gas volumes fed into the system correspond exactly to the respective uptake. The continuous measurement of oxygen uptake renders extensive monitoring of circulatory and metabolic functions possible.

Quantitative closed system anaesthesia is achieved only if the fresh gas composition and its volume correspond exactly to the patient's uptake. Only by this technique will it be possible to keep the anaesthetic gas composition and volume constant over the whole course of an anaesthetic, simultaneously dispensing completely with the discharge of any excess gas.

4.4   References

1. White, D C. Closed and low flow system anaesthesia. *Curr. Anaes. Crit. Care*, 3, 98–107 (1992)
2. Virtue, R. W. Minimal flow nitrous oxide anesthesia. *Anesthesiology*, **40**, 196–198 (1974)
3. Virtue, R. W. Toward closed system anesthesia. *Anaesthesist*, **26**, 545–546 (1977)
4. Foldes, F. F., Cervaolo, A. J. and Carpenter, S. L. The administration of nitrous oxide – oxygen anesthesia in closed systems. *Ann. Surg.*, **136**, 978–981 (1952)
5. Foldes, F. F. and Duncalf, D. Low flow anesthesia: a plea for simplicity. In *Alternative Methoden in der Anästhesie* (eds P. H. van Aken and U. Schneider), INA-Schriftenreihe, Bd. 50, Thieme, Stuttgart (1985), pp. 1–7
6. Grote, B., Adolphs, A. and Merten, G. Inhalationsnarkose im Low-Flow-System. In *Geschlossens System für Inhalationsnarkosen*, Internationales Symposium, Düsseldorf, 7–8 May, 1982 (Abstract)
7. Spieß, W. Narkose im geschlossenen System mit kontinuierlicher inspiratorischer Sauerstoffmessung. *Anaesthesist*, **26**, 503–513 (1977)
8. Spieß, W. Minimal-Flow Anästhesie – eine zeitgemäße Alternative für die Klinikroutine. *Anaesth. Reanim.*, **5**, 145–149 (1980)
9. Spieß, W. Sauerstoffverbrauch und Aufnahme von Lachgas und volatilen Anästhetika. In *Alternative Methoden in der Anästhesie* (eds P. Lawin, van Aken and U. Schneider), INA-Schriftenreihe, Bd. 50, Thieme, Stuttgart (1985), pp. 8–18
10. Baum, J. Klinische Anwendung der Minimal-Flow Anästhesie. In *Narkosebeatmung: Low Flow, Minimal flow, Geschlossenes System* (eds J.-P. A. H. Jantzen and P. P. Kleeman), Schattauer, Stuttgart (1989), pp. 49–66
11. Nunn, J. F. Techniques for induction of closed circuit anesthesia. In *Low Flow and Closed Circuit Anesthesia* (eds J. A. Aldrete, H. J. Lowe and R. W. Virtue), Grune and Stratton, New York (1979), pp. 3–10)
12. Deutsches Institut für Normung. *Deutsche Norm Inhalationsnarkosegeräte*, DIN 13 252. Beuth, Berlin (1984)
13. Barton, F. and Nunn, J. F. Totally closed circuit nitrous oxide/oxygen anaesthesia. *Br. J. Anaesth.*, **47**, 350–357 (1975)
14. Ernst, E. A. Closed circuit anesthesia. In *Refresher-Kurs ZAK 85* (eds F. W. List and H. V. Schalk), Akademische Druck- und Verlagsanstalt, Graz (1985)
15. Weingarten, M. Low flow and closed circuit anesthesia. In *Low Flow and Closed Circuit Anesthesia* (eds J. A. Aldrete, H. J. Lowe and R. W. Virtue), Grune and Stratton, New York (1979), pp. 67–74
16. Lowe, H. J. and Ernst, E. A. *The Quantitative Practice of Anesthesia*, Williams and Wilkins, Baltimore (1981)
17. White, D. C. Injection of liquid anaesthetic agents into breathing circuits. In *Geschlossenes System für Inhalationsnarkosen*, Internationales Symposium, Düsseldorf, 7–8 May, 1982 (Abstract)
18. Droh, R. Inhalationsnarkose im geschlossenen System. In *Geschlossenes System für Inhalationsnarkosen*, Internationales Symposium, Düsseldorff 7–8 May, 1982 (Abstract)
19. Wallroth, C. F. Technical conception for an anesthesia system with electronic metering of gases and vapors. *Acta Anaesth. Belg.*, **35**, 279–293 (1984)
20. Baum, J. Quantitative anaesthesia in the low-flow system. In *Quantitative Anaesthesia: Low Flow and Closed Circuit* (eds K. van Ackern, H. Frankenberger, E. Konecny and K. Steinbereithner), Anästhesiologie und Intensivmedizin, Bd. 204, Springer, Berlin (1989), pp. 44–57
21. Baum, J. Clinical applications of low flow and closed circuit anesthesia. *Acta Anaesth. Belg.*, **41**, 239–247
22. Westenskow, D. R. and Wallroth, C. F. Closed-loop control for anesthesia breathing systems. *J. Clin. Monit*, **6**, 249–256 (1990)
23. Wallroth, C. F., Jaklitsch, R. and Wied, H. A. Technical realisation of quantitative metering and ventilation. In *Quantitative Anaesthesia: Low Flow and Closed Circuit* (eds K. van

Ackern, H. Frankenberger, E. Konecny and K. Steinbereithner), Anästhesiologie und Intensivmedizin, Bd. 204. Springer, Berlin (1989), pp. 96–108

24. Erdmann, W., Veeger, A. I. and Verkaaik, A. P. K. Narkosebeatmungsgeräte: Gegenwart und Zukunft. In *Narkosebeatmung: Low Flow, Minimal flow, Geschlossenes System* (eds J.-P. A. H. and P. P. Kleemann), Schattauer, Stuttgart (1989), pp. 5–17

25. Versichelen, L. and Rolly, G. Mass-spectrometric evaluation of some recently introduced low flow, closed circuit systems. *Acta Anaesth. Belg.*, **41**, 225–237 (1990)

26. Waters, R. M. Clinical scope and utility of carbon dioxide filtration in inhalation anaesthesia. *Anesth. Analg*, **3**, 20–22 (1924)

Control of inhalational anaesthesia

The essential principles of anaesthesia management with reduced fresh gas flow can be demonstrated and rules for the control of inhalational anaesthesia established with the aid of computer simulations. Five computer programs for simulation of inhalational anaesthesia are discussed.

5.1 Computer simulation programs

5.1.1 Narkosesimulator

Narkosesimulator, developed by H. Schwilden, facilitates the simulation of concentration time courses of volatile anaesthetics in different tissues and organs as a function of dosage, parameters of the anaesthesia machine and ventilation, and anthropometric patient data[1]. Hardware requirements are an IBM PC or compatible computer, equipped with 256 kbyte RAM and a CGA graphics card. When using a computer with a Hercules graphic card, emulation of the CGA graphic mode can be effected by means of appropriate software (e.g. Vastscreen, Dawicontrol). Simulation can be displayed on a black-and-white screen, but a colour monitor is preferable. Simulation results can be printed out.

The assumed parameters of the anaesthesia machine and the patient on which simulation will be based are entered into the computer prior to simulation. This is the only currently available simulation program to permit variation of the breathing system volume. Regrettably, this program, produced in 1986, has never been updated. Simulation is started once the volatile anaesthetic halothane, enflurane, isoflurane or methoxyflurane has been selected and the fresh gas concentration assessed. The screen displays the concentration trends in a maximum of three preselected gas or tissue compartments.

The simulation, which is based on pharmacokinetic calculations, does not consider second-gas effects or biotransformation of the volatile anaesthetics. The calculations are based on the physiological relations of tissue composition and organ perfusion of adults, so that calculations for patients of less than 38 kg are not possible.

5.1.2   Gas Uptake Simulation

The program Gas Uptake Simulation, developed by Vanderlei et al.[2], facilitates the most extensive simulation with respect to changes of gas composition in the breathing system during the assumed performance of anaesthesia. Not only the concentration trends of the inhalational anaesthetics halothane, enflurane, isoflurane, methoxyflurane, ether and nitrous oxide are calculated, but also the concentrations of oxygen, nitrogen and carbon dioxide. The program comprises a tutorial and a two-part interactive teaching program, so that not only the handling of this software, but also the fundamentals and rules governing uptake and distribution of inhalational anaesthetics can be learned. This simulation program is also based only on pharmacokinetic algorithms – pharmacodynamic effects are not considered.

The program can be run with IBM compatible XT and AT computers featuring a RAM of at least 384 kbytes, which are equipped with two diskette drives or a hard disk. A CGA or Hercules graphics card is required. Furthermore, it requires the GEM user interface and operation is considerably simplified if use is made of a mouse. A later version of this program is available which runs under Microsoft Windows.

The data, the patient and machine parameters, plus the values for gas dosage, are selected and entered with pull-down menus and different windows. Depending on the screen selected, the simulation results are displayed numerically, or alternatively in a bar or a line graph, whereby the concentrations of six out of the 12 gas or tissue compartments can be displayed simultaneously. The GUS program enables the simultaneous simulation of two assumed anaesthesia courses, so that the changes in gas concentrations can be compared under different simulation conditions.

5.1.3   NARKUP

This program, developed by White and Lockwood[3], runs on IBM compatible computers with CGA, EGA, VGA or Hercules graphics card; a mathematics co-processor is supported.

Following selection of the breathing system, the values for the settings at the anaesthetic machine and the patient's parameters can be widely varied in accordance with the desired simulation. The calculated concentrations of nitrous oxide and volatile anaesthetics are displayed numerically at any time of simulation, while concentration trends are simultaneously displayed as a line graph during the simulation. In addition to simulation of anaesthesia with common anaesthetics, this program enables simulation with anaesthetics such as cyclopropane, sevoflurane, desflurane or xenon. Depending on the menu selected, the uptake of anaesthetics is displayed numerically as well as in a line graph.

5.1.4   Gas Man

The Gas Man simulation program, developed by Philip[4], runs with the 4.1 or later operating system on all Macintosh computers including Macintosh-Plus, SE and II series, which are equipped with 800 kbyte RAM. Alternatively, a Microsoft Windows version (Gas Man 2.0) is now available.

It is an interactive teaching program which explains the pharmacokinetic rules of uptake and distribution of volatile anaesthetics. The display is clear-cut and straightforward. Following selection of the breathing system, the values for fresh gas flow, alveolar ventilation and cardiac output are entered. The data can be varied during simulation. This program also not only simulates anaesthesia with common volatile anaesthetics but also with sevoflurane and desflurane. The gas concentrations in the gas-carrying compartment and in different tissues can be comprehensively displayed either in the form of a bargraph or as a line graph.

5.1.5   BODY Simulation

BODY Simulation (vers. β-3.1), developed by Ty Smith and coworkers[5], requires at least an IBM 486 DX or compatible computer (DX2 processor/ 66 MHz recommended, DX processor/33 MHz minimum), MS-DOS operating system version 5.0 or later, and 8 Mbyte RAM (4 Mbyte minimum). The program takes advantage of modern video technology; thus, a local bus SVGA card is recommended which has to be compatible with the VESA (Video Electronics Standards Association) standard. Since BODY Simulation incorporates various operating theatre sounds, the computer additionally should be equipped with a sound card. Sound Blaster, up to now, is the only fully supported audio card.

BODY Simulation is a computer-based trainer which simulates all functions of a fully equipped anaesthesia workstation and the reaction of the patient to ventilation and drug administration. The user can switch between a photorealistic view of the patient, a depiction of the machine's control panel, various different monitor displays, the screen for selection of currently 48 drugs and gases, and the screens displaying the results of simulation in different kinds of tables, time plots or bar graphs. Pressures, flows, resistances and compliances in the cardiovascular and pulmonary system, as well as gas or inhaled or injected agent concentrations in different tissues and gas containing compartments, can be analysed. BODY simulation is a very comprehensive tool, not only for educational purposes, but also for more experienced anaesthetists to improve not only their knowledge of the pharmacology and physiology of drugs, gases and vapours, but also the different functions of an anaesthetic machine. Scientifically orientated users may even create their own drugs or patients with specific physicochemical or physiological properties. The graphical trend displays of this beta release version, however, are not yet developed to commercial standards.

5.1.6   Clinical relevance of anaesthesia simulation by computer software

It must be admitted that most of the simulation programs are based upon simplified presuppositions:

- The oxygen consumption and the carbon dioxide production are assumed to be constant over the entire period of simulation, unless the preselected cardiac output has been changed.
- No consideration is given to the effects that changes in fluid balance (resulting from infusion or transfusion therapy or current loss of blood) have on the uptake and distribution of volatile anaesthetics.

- Loss of volatile anaesthetic by absorption in the breathing system's components, by diffusion via the skin and mucous membranes or by metabolism, are not given consideration in the calculations
- The solubility of volatile anaesthetic in blood and in tissues is assumed to be constant.
- The saturation of breathing gas with water vapour is assumed to be 100%.
- No consideration is given to the effects of temperature, haemoglobin content and pH blood value on the solubility of oxygen and carbon dioxide.
- Cardiac output, pulmonary and systemic shunt and dead space are assumed to be constant at the values entered at the beginning of simulation, unless they have subsequently been changed.
- Pharmacodynamic processes occurring during an inhalational anaesthesia are not considered during pharmacokinetic calculations.

It must be pointed out that, notwithstanding the complexity of pharmacokinetic algorithms, computer simulations are based on simplified process and compartment models. However, these programs are perfectly suited to illustration of the pharmacokinetics of uptake and distribution of volatile anaesthetics in a graphic manner. The great number of procedure, machine and patient-specific factors which affect the composition of anaesthetic gases in a breathing system can be illustrated individually via comparative simulations, so that their particular significance on anaesthetic management can be evaluated. To this end, simulation programs are not only a perfect teaching aid for the on-the-job training of physicians, but they also provide extensive information for experienced anaesthetists on the complex processes which determine the composition of anaesthetic gas in a breathing system. Only a sound understanding of the functions of anaesthesia machines and the interactions between patient and machine make it possible to use the currently available sophisticated anaesthetic technology to its full potential.

5.2   Control of inhalational anaesthesia

During the course of a surgical intervention, the concentration of the volatile anaesthetic, selected for inhalational anaesthesia, must be continuously adapted to the individual reactions and clinical requirements.

The anaesthetic concentration which is finally administered to the patient derives from a complex process which takes place in the breathing system, determined by a number of factors:

- by technical parameters such as the type of the breathing system, its technical design, the fresh gas utilization and the system's volume
- by the individual gas uptake of the patient which is determined by pharmacokinetic and pharmacodynamic characteristics
- by the selected fresh gas flow rate and the adjustment of the fresh gas composition, and
- by equipment-inherent conditions, such as the loss of anaesthetic gases or the entrance of air into the system as a result of leaks.

Therefore, the breathing system must not only be understood as being the technical conveyor of anaesthetic gases from the anaesthetic machine to the patient, it is also the essential interactive technical element by means of which the concentrations of anaesthetic gases are determined.

The following serves to explain to what extent the composition of anaesthetic gas is influenced by the fresh gas flow. This can clearly be demonstrated by means of computer simulation, since the fresh gas flow can be independently varied, while the remaining simulation conditions remain unchanged.

Unless otherwise specified, the following simulations are all based on identical simulation conditions. The breathing system used is a rebreathing system, the circle absorber system. The vaporizer is in the fresh gas supply (VOC). The volatile anaesthetic is isoflurane which is used on an adult patient of 75 kg body weight, with physiological circulatory conditions under normoventilation.

According to his own experience the author assumes that in the individual case the concentrations calculated by computer simulation may differ by about 10–15% from the values measured during clinical performance. Nevertheless, the simulated gas concentrations agree fairly well with the average values measured in larger clinical trials.

5.2.1   The induction phase

In the induction phase, a volatile anaesthetic is administered with the aim of obtaining an appropriate anaesthetic depth to permit commencement of a surgical intervention within an acceptable period of time. For this purpose, the desired anaesthetic concentration should not only be washed into the gas-carrying space, but also into the central nervous tissue.

In computer simulation of the induction phase (Figure 5.1a), the isoflurane concentration of the fresh gas is set to 1.5% at different fresh gas flows of 0.5, 1.0, 2.0 and 4.0 l/min. At lower fresh gas flows, the rise in the inspired isoflurane concentration is slower.

However, it is the end-tidal anaesthetic concentration which allows an estimate of the concentration in the blood and hence judgement of the depth of anaesthesia, since this corresponds approximately to the alveolar and thus arterial concentration[6]. With identical isoflurane concentration in the fresh gas, the rise in the expired anaesthetic concentration is similarly slower, the lower the fresh gas flow (Figure 5.1b).

If the intended expired isoflurane concentration is 0.8–0.9% – in addition to the MAC fraction of 60–70% of nitrous oxide, this corresponds approximately to the AD_{95} for isoflurane – this value can only be attained within an acceptably short initial period of 10–15 min with a fresh gas flow of 4 l/min.

This can be explained as follows (Figures 5.2a,b): with a given fresh gas flow of 4.0 l/min, the rebreathing volume is comparatively low, so that a high fresh gas portion is administered to the patient with each cycle. The isoflurane concentration of the inspired gas is therefore high. The alveolar–arterial partial pressure gradient is restored with each breath. This results in a high uptake which in turn leads to a fast increase in the expired isoflurane concentration.

On the other hand, with a low fresh gas flow of 0.5 l/min the rebreathing fraction increases considerably: the inspired isoflurane concentration is now

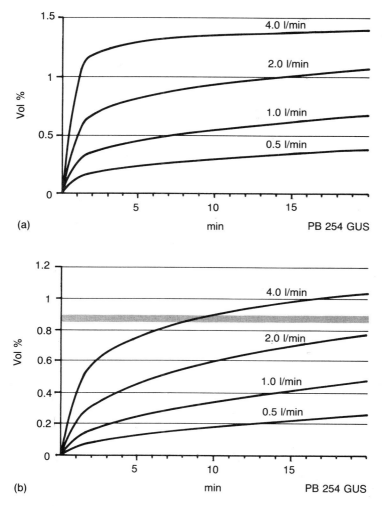

Figure 5.1 Induction phase: (a) inspired and (b) expired isoflurane concentration with different fresh gas flows, fresh gas isoflurane concentration 1.5%

almost exclusively determined by the composition of the isoflurane-depleted exhaled gas and increases only very slowly. The alveolar–arterial partial pressure gradient after each inspiration is thus low, as is the uptake, which in turn slows down the increase in the expired isoflurane concentration.

The increase in the expired anaesthetic concentration can be accelerated if, with the reduction of the fresh gas flow, the isoflurane concentration in the fresh gas is raised (Figure 5.3). The target concentration between 0.8% and 0.9% can thus be achieved within an approximately short period of time even with a fresh gas flow of only 1.0 l/min. However, this approach may not be practicable at a fresh gas flow of only 0.5 l/min, since the desired

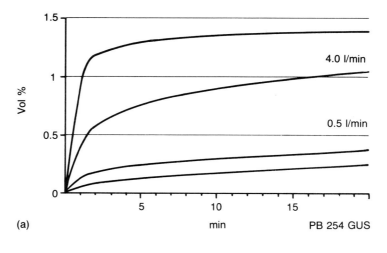

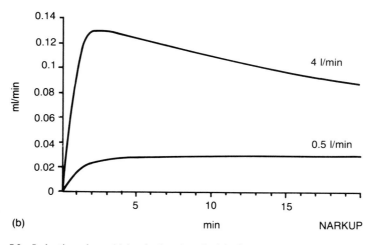

Figure 5.2 Induction phase: (a) inspired and expired isoflurane concentration with fresh gas flows of 4.0 versus 0.5 l/min, fresh gas isoflurane concentration 1.5%; (b) corresponding isoflurane uptake (ml liquid isoflurane)

concentration cannot be attained within an acceptable time if the output of the vaporizer is limited to 5%.

It is for this reason that, over a period of about 15 min, a rather high fresh gas flow – approximately 4 l/min – has to be selected for induction of anaesthesia, whereby the concentration of the anaesthetic in the fresh gas must be set approximately 0.5–1.0% higher than the target expired concentration. This is a reasonable way to increase the depth of inhalational anaesthesia within an appropriate period of time and to attain the desired anaesthetic gas composition.

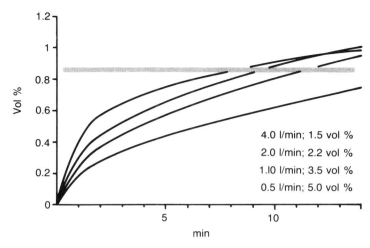

Figure 5.3 Induction phase: expired isoflurane concentration with different fresh gas flows
and differing isoflurane admixture

5.2.2   Maintenance of anaesthesia

5.2.2.1   *Adapting the fresh gas flow to the uptake*

Since, after completion of the induction phase, the uptake decreases
complementary to the increase in expired anaesthetic concentration, the fresh
gas flow can now be adapted to the reduced uptake. According to this concept
of minimal flow anaesthesia[7], Virtue recommends reducing the fresh gas flow
to 0.5 l/min after an induction phase of about 15 min. Only with an adequate
reduction of the fresh gas flow will it be possible to reduce the discharge of
excess gas from the system and thus to increase the rebreathing volume. This
is the only way to fully realize the advantages of rebreathing systems.

In another simulation (Figure 5.4), following a 15-minute induction phase
with a fresh gas flow of 4.5 l/min and fresh gas isoflurane concentration of
1.5%, the flow is reduced to 2.0, 1.0 or 0.5 l/min alternatively, while the
anaesthetic concentration is maintained. The greater the reduction of the
fresh gas flow, the greater the decrease in isoflurane concentration. This can
be attributed to the fact that the amount of anaesthetic vapour, which is
reduced to 30, 15 or even 7.5 ml/min as a result of flow reduction, is not able
to replenish the volume of isoflurane vapour which is taken up by the patient
or discharged with the excess gas.

However, if the isoflurane concentration is increased to 2.5% at the same
time as the fresh gas flow is reduced to 0.5 l/min, the target expired isoflurane
concentration of about 0.9% can be maintained in spite of an insignificant
initial decrease.

A standardized concept for control of inhalational anaesthesia according
to the Virtue scheme can thus be derived from the simulation results. During
the induction phase of 15–20 min, 1.5% isoflurane is added to a fresh gas
flow of 4.4 l/min. Following flow reduction to 0.5 l/min, the isoflurane

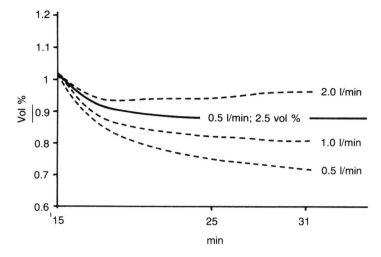

Figure 5.4   Expired isoflurane concentration after fresh gas flow reduction from 4.5 to 2.0, 1.0 or 0.5 l/min while fresh gas isoflurane concentration remained unchanged at 1.5%. For comparison: expired isoflurane concentration after fresh gas flow reduction from 4.5 to 0.5 l/min, with simultaneous increase of the isoflurane concentration from 1.5 to 2.5%

concentration is increased to 2.5%. An average expired isoflurane concentration of 0.85% can be attained with these standard settings. If such a dosage pattern is applied on a clinical trial, the measured anaesthetic concentrations correspond fairly well to the values predicted using computer simulation[8]. It should, however, be pointed out that these dosage schemes can only be regarded as guidelines for clinical practice. It goes without saying that this scheme has to be adjusted from case to case in line with individual variation and the clinical requirements.

5.2.2.2   Influence of the individual uptake

This is another characteristic of inhalational anaesthesia with low fresh gas flow that has considerable influence on the control of the volatile anaesthetic concentration (Figure 5.5a,b).

Due to the larger proportion of rebreathing, the gas concentration in the breathing system is affected to a larger extent by the composition of the exhaled gas, i.e. by the individual uptake, than is the case with a high fresh gas flow.

The uptake of heavyweight patients is greater than that of lightweight patients. This means that in minimal flow anaesthesia using an identical fresh gas concentration of 2.5% isoflurane, the expired isoflurane concentration of a 75 kg patient is lower than that of a 55 kg patient. Such differences in concentration were also observed in clinical trials on patients of different body weight[8]. With a comparatively high fresh gas flow of 4.4 l/min, however, the expired isoflurane concentration is only insignificantly influenced by the body weight of the patient (Figure 5.5a).

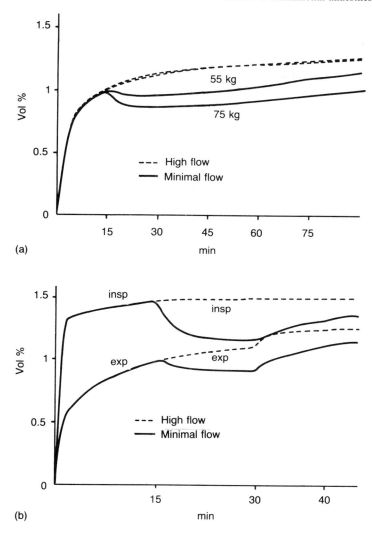

Figure 5.5 Concentration of the anaesthetic as a function of uptake: (a) expired isoflurane concentration as a function of body weight; (b) inspired and expired isoflurane concentration as a function of cardiac output

Furthermore, the individual uptake is correlated to the cardiac output. Once again, a computer simulated anaesthesia on a normal weight adult patient can be used as an illustration (Figure 5.5b). After 30 min of the simulation, the cardiac output is reduced by 50%, from 5.1 l/min to 2.5 l/min. While, under the conditions of anaesthesia with high flow, the inspired concentration does not change at all and expired concentration only insignificantly, there is a distinct increase in both the inspired and expired isoflurane concentration in anaesthesia with low fresh gas flow.

5.2.3   The time constant

The fact that the inertia of the system increases considerably with reduction of the fresh gas flow will be demonstrated by means of comparison between high flow and minimal flow anaesthesia (Figure 5.6a,b).

For anaesthesia with high fresh gas flow, the flow remains constant at 4.4 l/min over the entire period of anaesthesia. During the first 25 min, an isoflurane concentration of 1.5% is set at the vaporizer. The clinical situation

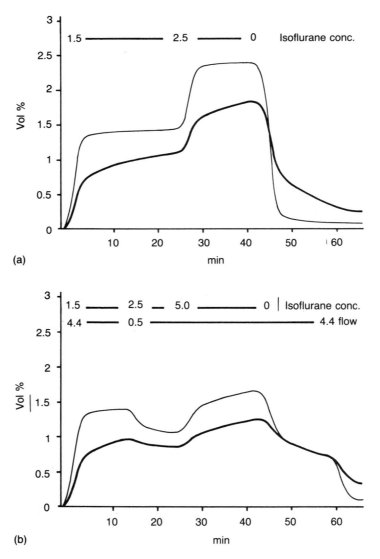

Figure 5.6   Time constants for comparison: high flow anaesthesia (4.4 l/min) versus minimal flow anaesthesia

at that time calls for an increase of the anaesthetic depth and so the isoflurane concentration in the fresh gas is increased to 2.5%. After 40 min, the vaporizer is switched off.

In this example of high flow anaesthesia, the changes in the fresh gas concentration result in a rapid change in inspired and expired anaesthetic concentration in the breathing system.

During the initial phase of the minimal flow anaesthetic which is shown for comparison, an isoflurane concentration of 1.5% is set with a fresh gas flow of 4.4 l/min. With reduction of the flow to 0.5 l/min, the isoflurane concentration in the fresh gas is increased to 2.5%. In spite of the insignificant decrease in inspired and expired anaesthetic concentration, the latter stabilizes at the target value of between 0.8% and 0.9%. In this example, the clinical situation also calls for an increase of the anaesthetic depth after 25 min. While maintaining the low flow, the vaporizer is therefore set to its maximum output of 5% isoflurane, and switched off again after 40 min.

In the case of minimal flow anaesthesia, even drastic changes of the fresh gas concentration will cause only delayed and slow changes of the inspired and expired anaesthetic concentrations in the breathing system.

Quantitatively, this phenomenon can be determined by calculation of the time constant T, which is a measure for that time in which concentration changes in the fresh gas result in corresponding concentration changes in the breathing system. According to Conway[9], the time constant can be calculated by the division of the system's volume (V_S) by the difference between fresh gas flow ($\dot{V}_F$) and uptake ($\dot{V}_U$):

$$T = V_S/(\dot{V}_F - \dot{V}_U) \ (\text{min})$$

This means that with a given uptake and given system volume, the time constant of a breathing system is inversely proportional to the fresh gas flow.

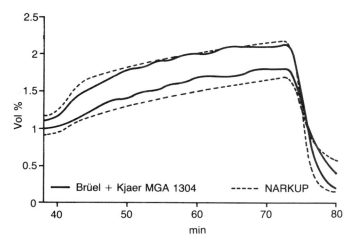

Figure 5.7   The long time constant of minimal flow anaesthesia in a clinical example (patient aged 41 years, weight 76 kg, height 1.79 m). At 40 min, the isoflurane fresh gas concentration is increased to 5%. After 75 min, the system is flushed with pure oxygen (4 l/min)

As a numerical value, the time constant quantifies the speed of wash-in and wash-out processes. After time T has passed, the anaesthetic concentration in the breathing system attains 63% of the final concentration, after $2 \times T$ 86.5% and after $3 \times T$ about 93%. Assuming a system volume of 5 litres, a functional residual capacity of 2.5 litres and a current uptake of 0.35 l/min, the following time constants can be calculated as a function of the fresh gas flow. $T = 39.2$ s at 8.0 l/min fresh gas flow, 2.0 min at 4.0 l/min, 4.5 min at 2.0 l/min, 11.5 min at 1.0 l/min and 50 min at 0.5 l/min. These extended time constants have to be borne in mind during the use of low flow techniques.

The long time constant of a rebreathing system used with low fresh gas flow is verified by another clinical example (Figure 5.7). A minimal flow anaesthetic was undertaken on a male patient (aged 41, weight 76 kg, height 179 cm), according to the standardized dosing scheme. After 40 min, the isoflurane concentration in the fresh gas was increased to 5% while the flow of 0.5 l/min was maintained. During the following 30 min, both the inspired and expired isoflurane concentration (measured by means of a Brüel and Kjaer gas analyser MGA 1304) rose only very slowly, in accordance with the long time constant. The correspondence between the values calculated by computer simulation and the actually measured concentrations is once more convincingly demonstrated in this example.

5.2.4   Emergence from anaesthesia

The emergence phase of anaesthesia is aimed at a rapid reduction of anaesthetic depth until the patient wakes up. The anaesthetic concentration in the breathing system should therefore be rapidly reduced (Figure 5.8a,b).

Following an anaesthetic of 45 min duration with high fresh gas flow and an isoflurane concentration of 1.5%, the vaporizer is switched off and the system flushed with oxygen flows of 0.5, 1.0, 2.0 and 4.0 l/min. As can be expected in accordance with the respective time constants, the expired isoflurane concentration decreases more slowly with the lower oxygen flows (Figure 5.8a).

If the system is flushed with a high oxygen flow of 4.0 l/min, the rebreathing proportion is comparatively low and the inspired oxygen tension correspondingly high. The high alveolar–capillary partial pressure gradient causes a rapid discharge of the anaesthetic and a correspondingly rapid decrease in the expired isoflurane concentration (Figure 5.8b).

5.3   Characteristics of anaesthesia management as a function of fresh gas flow

According to their intended use, rebreathing systems can be operated with either high or low fresh gas flows[10]. The advantages of rebreathing can only be realized provided that during the course of anaesthesia the fresh gas flow is adapted to the uptake. However, in varying the flow, the characteristic of the breathing system, i.e. the dynamics of volatile anaesthetic administration, may be subject to considerable changes.

With a high fresh gas flow, the composition of the anaesthetic gas corresponds approximately to that of the fresh gas. The greater portion of

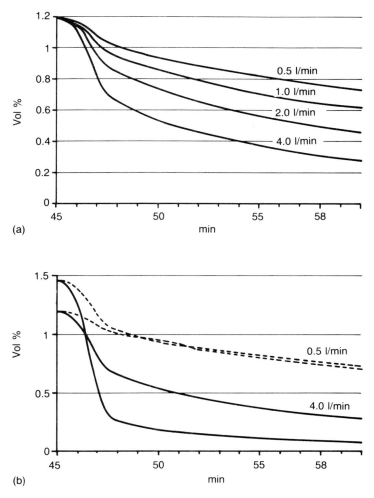

Figure 5.8 Emergence phase: (a) expired isoflurane concentration at different flows of pure oxygen; (b) inspired and expired isoflurane concentration during flushing of the system with pure oxygen at 4.0 versus 0.5 l/min

the exhaled gas is discharged via the waste valve; the rebreathing fraction is insignificant. Since a high fresh gas portion is insufflated into the lungs with each ventilation stroke, a high alveolar–arterial partial pressure gradient, which is essentially determined by the fresh gas composition, is newly re-established with each breath. This results in an accelerated gas exchange between the gas and the blood compartment and a correspondingly rapid wash-in and wash-out of the anaesthetic. Only if the partial pressures between alveolar and blood compartment are balanced will the uptake or discharge of the volatile anaesthetic decrease in accordance with the lower partial pressure gradient.

On the other hand, the discharge of excess gas volume from the system decreases with a low fresh gas flow. The greater part of the exhaled gas remains in the system, is mixed with the small fresh gas volume and is routed back to the patient during the next inspiration. The composition of the anaesthetic gas is thus essentially determined by the composition of exhaled gas. But approximately 85% of the exhaled breath consists of alveolar gas. This means that in previous ventilation cycles the partial pressures of this gas have already been aligned to those of the blood compartment. The partial pressure gradient between the alveolar and blood compartments established with each inspiration is accordingly low, and the same has to be assumed for the uptake or discharge of the volatile anaesthetic.

5.4   Rules on anaesthetic management

Whenever the concentration of the anaesthetic in the gas-carrying compartment is to be rapidly increased or reduced, that is if short time constants have to be used, the fresh gas flow has to be set to comparatively high values. The setting of the anaesthetic fresh gas concentration may then be closer to the target inspired concentration.

But whenever anaesthesia has reached the desired depth, and the uptake has reached low values in steady state of anaesthesia, long time constants, i.e. low fresh gas flow, can be used. The difference between the fresh gas anaesthetic concentration and the intended inspired concentration has to be assumed to be greater at lower fresh gas flows.

If, while maintaining a low fresh gas flow, the anaesthetic is to be deepened or lightened, the concentration in the fresh gas must be adjusted to values distinctly above or below the target inspired concentration. The composition of the inspired gas will differ distinctly from that of the expired gas only if the amount of anaesthetic fed into the system by the low fresh gas volume is sufficiently increased or reduced. The resulting high alveolar–capillary partial pressure gradient will enhance the gas exchange between the gas and the blood compartment. It must be considered, though, that, as the output of the vaporizers is limited, this procedure is subject to distinct limitation as a function of the fresh gas flow selected.

5.5   References

1. Schwilden, H. Narkosesimulator, Deutsche Abbott, Wiesbaden (1986)
2. Vanderlei, P., Spain, J. and Thompson, K. Gas Uptake Simulation, PB GUS (Vers. PB 3.0), Puritan-Bennett Corporation, 9401 Indian Creek, Bld. 40, Suite 300, Overland Park, KS 66 210 (1987)
3. White, D. C. and Lockwood, G. Narkup (Vers. 4.11), Northwick Park Hospital and Clinical Research Centre, Harrow, Middlesex HA1 3UJ (1989)
4. Philip, J. A. Gas Man. Med Man Simulations, P.O. box 67-160, Chestnut Hill, MA 02167 (1991)
5. Charbonneau, P., Davidson, T., Duranteau, R., Soukup, P., Starko, K., Starkom S. and Ty Smith, N. BODY Simulation, Advanced Simulation Corporation, 18002 Cowan, Suite 201E, Irvine, CA 92714, USA (1994)

6. Zbinden, A. M. Inhalationsanästhetika: Aufnahme und Verteilung, Wissenschaftliche Verlagsabteilung, Deutsche Abbott, Wiesbaden (1987)
7. Virtue, R. W. Minimal flow nitrous oxide anesthesia. *Anesthesiology*, **40**, 196–198 (1974)
8. Baum, J. Klinische Anwendung der Minimal-Flow-Anästhesie. In *Narkosebeatmung. Low Flow, Minimal Flow, Geschlossenes System* (eds J. P. A. H. Jantzen and P. P. Kleeman) Schattauer, Stuttgart (1989), pp. 49–66
9. Conway, C. M. Closed and low flow systems. Theoretical considerations. *Acta Anaesth. Belg.*, **34**, 257–263 (1984)
10. Bergmann, H. Das Narkosegerät in Gegenwart und Zukunft aus der Sicht des Klinikers. *Anaesthesist*, **35**, 587–594 (1986)

Advantages of rebreathing

6.1 Reduced consumption of anaesthetic gases

The extent to which the consumption of anaesthetic gases can be reduced by appropriate reduction of the fresh gas flow will be explained by the example of minimal flow anaesthesia. During performance of an isoflurane anaesthetic on a 75 kg patient, the fresh gas volume is reduced to 0.5 l/min after an initial 15-minute phase with high flow of 4.4 l/min. The duration of anaesthesia is assumed to be 2 h and the target expired isoflurane concentration is about 1.0%. This minimal flow anaesthetic will be compared with an anaesthetic of identical duration and identical anaesthetic concentration, but with the high flow of 4.4 l/min maintained throughout. In this example, the total nitrous oxide consumption is reduced by 294 litres, oxygen consumption by 115.5 litres, and the consumption of isoflurane vapour by 5.62 litres (Figure 6.1). In longer lasting anaesthetics, the reduction of the anaesthetic gas consumption will be all the more pronounced.

Between 1984 and 1989, P. Feiss made a consistent switch in his clinic from non-rebreathing systems to rebreathing systems used with low fresh gas flow. In spite of a 25% increase in the number of anaesthetics undertaken, the annual nitrous oxide consumption could be reduced by about 40% from 9200 kg to 5880 kg. With this drastic change in management, the isoflurane consumption could even be reduced by 90–93%[1].

Comparing high flow (breathing system: Mapleson D) with low flow (circle absorber system) isoflurane–nitrous oxide anaesthesia, Pedersen[2] found, in procedures lasting 2 h, mean isoflurane consumptions of 40.8 ml and 7.9 ml, respectively. A 54.7% reduction in the consumption of isoflurane and a 55.9% reduction in that of enflurane are reported by Cotter[3]. He made his investigation in entirely unselected clinical trials. The fresh gas flows compared were about 6.5 l/min in the 'high flow' group, but were only a little below 3 l/min and somewhat inconsistent in the 'low flow' group.

In Germany, about 5 million anaesthetic procedures are performed each year, and in the UK, about 3.5 million[4]. If it is assumed that 20% are regional blocks, 20% total intravenous techniques or operations of short duration, in which low flow anaesthesia would not be practical, then there are potential savings to be made in over 5 million cases in these two countries alone. Let us assume that enflurane is used in 50% of these cases, and isoflurane in the remaining 50%, and that the average end-expiratory concentration is 0.8

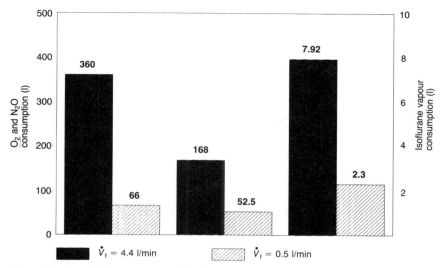

Figure 6.1   Anaesthetic gas consumption in litres over a period of 120 min. High flow anaesthesia ($\dot{V}_f$:4.4 l/min) versus minimal flow anaesthesia ($\dot{V}_f$:0.5 l/min)

Table 6.1   Estimation of annual anaesthetic gas consumption and reduction of costs which could result from concomitant changes from high to low flow anaesthesia in Germany and the UK*

	Consumption (l/year) (Fresh gas flow rate 4.5 l/min)	Consumption (l/year) (Fresh gas flow rate 1.0 l/min)	Cost savings (US$/year)
Oxygen	700×10^6	350×10^6	510 000
N$_2$O	1.5×10^9	0.5×10^9	12 200 000
Isoflurane	61 650	28 500	31 800 000
Enflurane	89 500	43 250	20 850 000

*Values for isoflurane and enflurane represent volume of liquid[4].

MAC. Let us presume also that 50% of these anaesthetics last for 1 h, 33% for 2 h and 17% for 3 h. It would be common practice in each case to use a fresh gas flow rate of 4.5 l/min for a total of 30 min, so as to facilitate wash-in and wash-out of the anaesthetic gases at appropriate times. If, under these preconditions, a low flow technique (1 l/min) is compared with a high flow anaesthesia (4.5 l/min), the reduction of gas and anaesthetic consumption can be projected to be about 350 million litres of oxygen, 1.000 million litres of nitrous oxide, 33 000 litres of liquid isoflurane and 46 000 litres of liquid enflurane per year (Table 6.1).

6.2   Reduced costs

6.2.1   Anaesthetic gases

It is self-evident that reduction of anaesthetic gas consumption is accompanied by a reduction of costs. Based on the previous example of a 2-hour isoflurane anaesthetic, performed according to the standardized scheme used routinely in the author's own hospital, the reduction of the fresh gas flow from 4.4 l/min to 0.5 l/min results in cost savings of 72.4%, which means that about 33.90 DM (22.60 US$) can be saved. Based on the German prices for anaesthetic gases, approximately 83.7% of the savings can be attributed to the reduction of isoflurane consumption, 15.6% to that of nitrous oxide and only 0.7% to the reduction of oxygen consumption (Figure 6.2). The cost savings depend on the duration of the anaesthetic procedure and the price of the agent selected (Figure 6.3) and of course, on the extent of flow reduction (Figure 6.4).

The different calculations concerning the saving of costs by flow reduction[2,3,5,6], are hardly comparable as all are based on quite different assumptions. Nevertheless, if an attempt is made to compile the different results, depending on the extent of flow reduction and the choice of the anaesthetic agent, a saving in costs due to reduced anaesthetic gas consumption of between 50% and 75% may be assumed for 1 h of anaesthesia

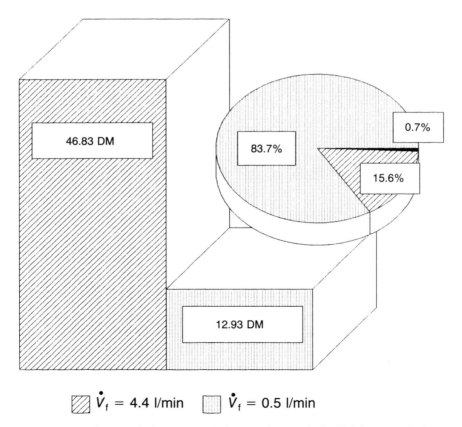

$\dot{V}_f$ = 4.4 l/min $\dot{V}_f$ = 0.5 l/min

Figure 6.2   Costs for anaesthetic gases used during 120 min anaesthesia. High flow anaesthesia (4.4 l/min) versus minimal flow anaesthesia (0.5 l/min). Pie chart indicates the breakdown of cost savings: isoflurane 83.7%, nitrous oxide 15.6%, oxygen 0.7%

(Table 6.2). Several authors emphasize that, in calculating the real costs of anaesthesia, the expenses for the soda lime, the supplementary intravenous drugs, the choice of the breathing system, expenses for acquisition and maintenance of the equipment, and last but not least the staff salaries, have also to be considered. Although the arguments are quite justified, these

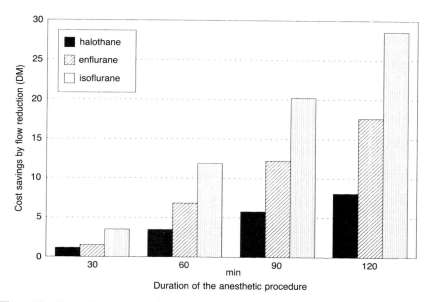

Figure 6.3   Cost savings by flow reduction as a function of duration of procedure and choice of anaesthetic agent

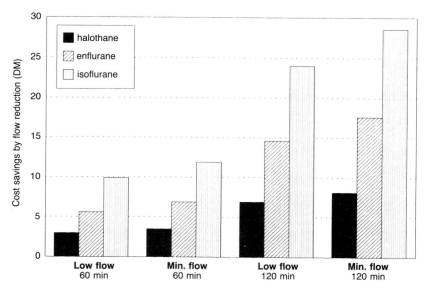

Figure 6.4   Cost savings as a function of degree of flow reduction

Table 6.2   Costs for anaesthetic gases as a function of the fresh gas flow (1 h anaesthesia)*

	$\simeq 6\,l/min$	$\simeq 4\,l/min$	$\simeq 3\,l/min$	$\simeq 1\,l/min$
Baum[5]				
isoflurane		28.50 DM		11.20 DM
		19.00 US$		7.47 US$
enflurane		18.00 DM		8.30 DM
		12.00 US$		5.53 US$
Cotter et al.[3]				
isoflurane	£11.40		£5.16	
	17 US$		7.70 US$	
enflurane	£5.62		£2.48	
	8.40 US$		3.70 US$	
Loke et al.[6]				
isoflurane	12 $Aus		6 $Aus	2 $Aus
	8 US$		4 US$	1.30 US$
enflurane	8.64 $Aus		4.30 $Aus	1.44 $Aus
	5.80 US$		2.90 US$	0.96 US$
Pedersen et al.[2]				
isoflurane	107 DKK		48.50 DKK	21 DKK
	14.50 US$		6.50 US$	2.90 US$

*DM, German Mark; US$, US dollar; £, pound Sterling; $Aus, Australian dollar; DKK, Danish kroner.

factors, except the soda lime consumption, are not directly linked to the setting of the fresh gas flow. One must not forget that every day many anaesthetic procedures are performed with technically advanced anaesthetic machines equipped with rebreathing systems and comprehensive monitoring, but using fresh gas flows which surely prevent the occurrence of any rebreathing. A more efficient use of available equipment by changing clinical practice alone would result in considerable savings.

Cost savings of between 55% and 75%[5,7] appear to be absolutely realistic if minimal flow anaesthesia is used consistently. Ernst has compared the cost involved in anaesthesia management with non-rebreathing systems with those in which closed rebreathing systems were used. If 10000 anaesthetics are performed with rebreathing systems (60% of 1 h, 30% of 2 h and 10% of 3 h), this results in cost savings of 6930 US$ if halothane is used, 36670 US$ for enflurane and 63560 US$ if isoflurane is used[8]. Cotter[3] comes to the conclusion, that routine use of low flow anaesthesia (4–3 l/min!) could result in annual savings of £26870 at his hospital, and Matjasko[9] reported annual savings of about 16800 US$ by performance of isoflurane anaesthesia using low flow at his department. Herscher and Yeakel estimated that, in 1977, the financial loss in the USA, resulting from the unnecessary discharge of unused excess gas out of breathing systems, added up to about 80 million US$[10]. For an average procedure such as a cholecystectomy, the costs involved for a neurolept anaesthesia with non-rebreathing system, for an enflurane anaesthesia via a semi-closed rebreathing system with a fresh gas flow of about 4 l/min, and for minimal flow anaesthesia with isoflurane are almost identical[11].

If the preconditions detailed in Section 6.1 are assumed, the annual financial savings resulting from reduced gas and anaesthetic consumption in Germany and the UK would total more than 65.4 million US$ if low flow anaesthetic techniques were performed consistently (Table 6.1). In addition, the efficiency of fresh gas utilization, i.e. the cost/benefit ratio of an anaesthetic method, can be described by the quotient of uptake and fresh gas volume:

$$Q_{eff} = \dot{V}_u / \dot{V}_f$$

where Q_{eff} = efficiency quotient
$\dot{V}_u$ = uptake
$\dot{V}_f$ = amount of gas contained in the fresh gas.

This quotient, thus, has to be calculated separately for nitrous oxide, oxygen and the volatile anaesthetic[8]. If the fresh gas flow and composition are kept constant, it is self-explanatory that during the course of anaesthesia the efficiency quotient varies with changes in uptake. The values established in a comparison between an anaesthetic with a high fresh gas flow of 4.4 l/min and a minimal flow anaesthetic of a normal-weight adult patient over a period of 30 min after induction are illustrated in Table 6.3.

The efficiency of fresh gas utilization increases considerably with reduction of the fresh gas flow. This quotient for oxygen, nitrous oxide and the volatile anaesthetic can only reach its maximum value of 1 in the case of quantitative closed system anaesthesia.

An ether structure and halogenation exclusively by fluorine are the characteristics of the newer volatile anaesthetics such as desflurane. The molecular structure of this agent results in low solubility and low anaesthetic potency. Its pharmacokinetic and pharmacodynamic properties result in a low uptake, although a comparatively high alveolar partial pressure must be established and maintained. If high flow anaesthesia is performed, most of the exhaled anaesthetic is vented to the atmosphere. Thus most of the inhaled anaesthetic is wasted, and the corresponding high amount of agent which has to be delivered into the system is needed only to re-establish the required high alveolar concentration and not to meet a high uptake. By contrast, using a low flow system, the low uptake of desflurane may even permit a reduction in the anaesthetic fresh gas concentration because it will be necessary only to supply a volume equivalent to the small amount of

Table 6.3 Efficiency quotient*

Fresh gas flow:	4.4 l/min	0.5 l/min
Fresh gas composition	32% O_2, 68% N_2O	60% O_2, 40% N_2O
	1.1 vol% isoflurane	2.3 vol% isoflurane
	3.5 vol% desflurane	3.5 vol% desflurane
Isoflurane	0.23	0.96
Desflurane	0.09	0.79
Oxygen	0.18	0.85
Nitrous oxide	0.06	0.91

*Uptake 30 min after induction (target exp. isoflurane concentration 0.85%, target exp. desflurane concentration 3.2%, weight of patient 75 kg): isoflurane 11.1 ml/min, desflurane 11.7 ml/min, O_2 254.9 ml/min, N_2O 182.6 ml/min.

vapour which is being taken up by the patient, together with a small volume equivalent to that vented to the atmosphere. The lower the solubility and the lower the anaesthetic potency of an anaesthetic agent, the higher will be the increase in efficiency which can be gained by flow reduction[4].

The greater economy of anaesthesia methods with reduced fresh gas flow cannot be denied. However, it must be emphasized that these techniques can only be considered as being advantageous provided that they are just as safe for the patient as methods performed with high fresh gas flows.

6.2.2 Soda lime consumption

In a number of publications it was assumed that the savings in anaesthetic gases resulting from flow reduction were offset by increased soda lime consumption[12,13]. In calculating the costs involved for low flow anaesthesia, only a few publications gave consideration to the costs for increased soda lime consumption, whereby calculations were based on theoretically derived carbon dioxide production and the soda lime's absorption capacity. With a consistent reduction of the fresh gas flow to 0.5 l/min, the costs for soda lime should increase by a factor of 3–7[11,13,14].

However, under clinical conditions, the actual consumption of soda lime by carbon dioxide absorption is not only influenced by the fresh gas flow, but by many other factors too, which can hardly be comprehensively included in the calculation. These include individual metabolic variations (net carbon dioxide production), ventilation and equipment parameters (fresh gas utilization), and the type, frequency and duration of the anaesthetic procedures.

In my own department the absorption capacity of soda lime was measured under clinical conditions with different fresh gas flows of 4.4 and 0.5 l/min using various anaesthetic machines: AV 1, Cicero and Sulla 800 V (Drägerwerk AG, Lübeck)[5,15]. The AV 1 and Sulla 800 V were equipped with an absorber canister of 1 litre volume and the Cicero with an absorber of 1.5 litres capacity and pelleted soda lime (ICI-Pharma, Plankstadt) was used. Consideration has to be given to the fact that, depending on the duration of anaesthesia and frequency of surgical interventions on an unselected patient group, it was by no means possible to work with a flow of 0.5 l/min at all times. The flow had to be increased for the induction and emergence phases, and a number of procedures, such as anaesthesia using a face mask, cannot be performed with reduced flow. This means that, prior to evaluation of the results, an accurate analysis had to be established to assess the percentage of time during which a fresh gas flow of 0.5 l/min was actually used. Soda lime was considered as being exhausted if the inspired carbon dioxide concentration had reached a value of 1%.

If a fresh gas flow of 4.4 l/min was used exclusively, the utilization time, until soda lime was completely exhausted, amounted to 99 h (Cicero), 62 h (AV 1) or 43 h (Sulla 800 V). Based on the current German price of 7.25 DM ($\simeq 4.83$ US$) per litre soda lime, the costs involved for soda lime under these conditions range between 0.11 DM ($\simeq 0.07$ US$) (Cicero) and 0.17 DM ($\simeq 0.13$ US$) (Sulla 800 V) per hour of anaesthesia.

If, whenever possible, the fresh gas flow was reduced to 0.5 l/min, the time of minimal flow anaesthesia with respect to total anaesthetic time ranged

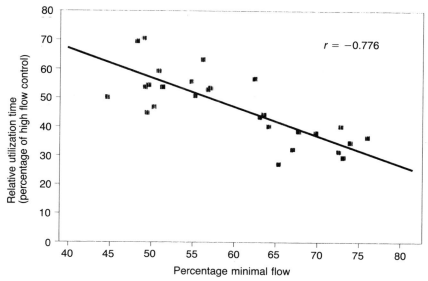

Figure 6.5   Utilization time of soda lime (depicted as percentage of utilization time, using a flow of 4.4 l/min), as a function of the percentage of time, during which anaesthesia was actually performed with 0.5 l/min fresh gas flow

between 45% and 75%. The time during which anaesthesia can actually be performed with a low fresh gas flow essentially depends on the duration and the frequency of anaesthetic procedures. Even if a large proportion of anaesthetics are of long duration and reduction of the fresh gas flow is effected consistently, the share that minimal flow phases have in the entire time of absorber operation under clinical conditions can hardly be extended above 75–85%. The utilization time of soda lime up to complete exhaustion is then reduced to 20–30% of the utilization period measured for a fresh gas flow of 4.4 l/min (Figure 6.5).

Thus, with the greatest possible use of minimal flow anaesthesia, the costs for soda lime rise by a factor of four. With a view to the earlier example of a 2 h isoflurane anaesthetic, this means that the costs for soda lime rise from 0.30 DM ($\simeq$ 0.20 US\$) to about 1.20 DM ($\simeq$ 0.80 US\$). Compared with the savings in anaesthetic gases which amount to 33.90 DM ($\simeq$ 22.60 US\$), the additional costs for soda lime, about 0.90 DM ($\simeq$ 0.60 US\$), are insignificant. The same conclusion was reached by Cotter[3].

6.3   Reduced environmental pollution

6.3.1   Workplace exposure to anaesthetic gas

Although neither harmfulness nor harmlessness of sub-anaesthetic gas concentrations have yet been demonstrated[16,17], workplace exposure to anaesthetic gases is gaining more importance with growing environmental awareness. In the USA, the following threshold limit values have been assessed by the National Institute of Occupational Safety and Health (NIOSH): for nitrous oxide 25 ppm, for all volatile anaesthetics 2 ppm, and for all volatile anaesthetics used together with nitrous oxide 0.5 ppm[8,18]. The TLV list (Table of Threshold Limit Values) assesses a value of 50 ppm for nitrous oxide and for halothane, and 75 ppm ($= 575 \, mg/m^3$) for enflurane.

Where the newest German MAK value list 1994 (MAK = Maximale Arbeitsplatz-Konzentration = maximum workplace concentration) is concerned, halothane is listed with a MAK of $40 \, mg/m^3$ ($= 5$ ppm) and nitrous oxide with 100 ppm[19]. The authorities for occupational safety and health in different German states countries specified MAK values for enflurane and isoflurane at $77 \, mg/m^3$ ($= 10$ ppm) within their area of responsibility[16]. In the Instructions on Handling of Anaesthetic Gases, issued by the Authority for Occupational Safety and Health in Hamburg, as of August 1990 the limit value for nitrous oxide has even been assessed at $91 \, mg/m^3$ ($= 50$ ppm)[20].

Virtue[21] proved that only by reduction of the nitrous oxide flow to 0.5 or 0.2 l/min the nitrous oxide workplace concentration could be reduced to 29 or 15 ppm, respectively (Figure 6.6). These values would even satisfy the stringent NIOSH requirements. As far as intubation anaesthesia is concerned, minimizing of emissions according to the 'state of the art', as is also sought by the German national regulations on harmful substances, could be realized on its own only by means of adequate reduction of the fresh gas flow and judicious use of rebreathing systems.

It is obvious that workplace contamination with anaesthetic gases can be considerably reduced by the use of gas scavenging systems, so that this

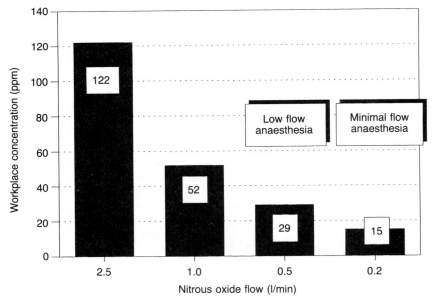

Figure 6.6   Reduction of workplace contamination with nitrous oxide by reduction of nitrous oxide flow. At a flow of 0.2 l/min (minimal flow anaesthesia), the value falls below the stringent NIOSH threshold (From Virtue[21], by permission)

problem is essentially overcome. However, it must be considered that at present the anaesthetic waste gases are discharged into the atmosphere.

6.3.2 Reduction of atmospheric pollution

6.3.2.1 Nitrous oxide

Every year the nitrous oxide concentration in the troposphere increases by 0.25%. This gas contributes to the continuous warming of the atmosphere, the so-called 'greenhouse effect'[22]. Nitrous oxide molecules are extremely stable. During their lifetime of some 150 years they may ascend up to the stratosphere and being involved in the destruction of the ozone layer by generating nitric oxides (Figure 6.7)[18,23]. However, it also must be considered that vastly more nitrous oxide is generated in fertilized agricultural soil by bacterial nitrate decomposition. Less than 1% of the emitted volume of nitrous oxide is estimated to derive from medical sources[22,24].

6.3.2.2 Halogenated hydrocarbons

Volatile anaesthetics like halothane, enflurane and isoflurane belong to the chlorofluorocarbon (CFC) group, which is held to be mainly responsible for the destruction of the ozone layer[22,23]. But the chlorofluorocarbons used as inhalational anesthetics are only partially substituted; that is, not all valencies of the carbon atoms are occupied by halogens. According to the ozone convention of Vienna and the protocol of Montreal, these partially substituted chlorofluorocarbons are held to be less noxious, as the ozone-destroying

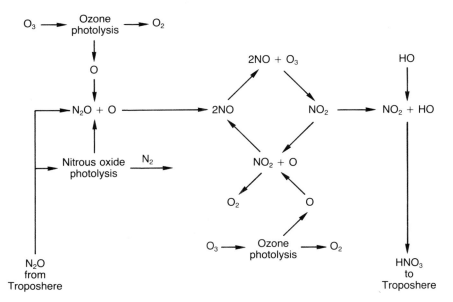

Figure 6.7   The reaction of nitrous oxide with stratospheric ozone (From Waterson[18], by permission)

potential is less than 5% of that exerted by fully substituted molecules[25]. Furthermore, these molecules have a comparatively short lifetime of about 2–6 years and are thus already being destroyed in the troposphere[22,26,27]. Last but not least, the quantity of volatile anaesthetics is estimated to be not more than 0.1% of the yearly production of industrially used CFCs[22,25]. However, it has to be considered critically that the figures describing the quantity of yearly global volatile agent production range widely from 100 tons[25] to 6400 tons[27]. The same criticism applies to the quoted figures for the amount of industrially produced and emitted CFCs, which differ considerably between publications. Thus, for the time being it seems to be nearly impossible to quantify exactly the contribution that the emission of volatile anaesthetics exerts on the destruction of the ozone layer[28].

Even though atmospheric pollution occurs with anaesthetic gases, their contribution to the greenhouse effect and the destruction of the ozone layer seem to be of minor importance. However, any environmental contamination with inhalation anaesthetics should be avoided conscientiously[22,27,29]. This goal seems to be all the more justified, as environmental pollution with anaesthetic gases can be considerably reduced simply by the judicious use of the available modern, technically advanced rebreathing systems[18,22,24].

6.4   Improved anaesthetic gas climate

In terms of clinical relevance, the anaesthetic gas climate can be improved if the share of cold dry fresh gas is reduced, while at the same time the proportion of recirculating humidified and warmed exhales gas is increased[30,31].

The significance that appropriate humidification and warming of anaesthetic gases have on the function of the ciliated epitheleum, i.e. mucociliary clearance, has been convincingly proved. Given a relative humidity of 50% for inspired gas at room temperature, a cessation of ciliary movement can already be observed 10 min after commencement of ventilation. Considerable morphological damage to the epithelium of the respiratory tract is caused by 3 h of ventilation with dry gases. Together with the drying up of secretions, which results from inadequate humidification and warming up of the inspired gas, this leads to mucus retention with partial obstruction of the bronchioles, which in turn supports the development of microatelectases. In addition, the improvement of the tracheobronchial climate helps in reducing fluid and heat loss via the respiratory tract.

During anaesthetic ventilation, the absolute humidity of the inspired gas should preferably range between 17 and 30 mg H_2O/l, and the breathing gas temperature between 28°C and 32°C[32–34].

Climatization of breathing gases is determined by the technical design of the breathing system, the size of the absorber, length and heat conduction of patient hoses, the ambient temperature, ventilation patterns and the fresh gas flow, i.e. the extent of rebreathing. This explains why a great number of investigations were carried out at quite different starting conditions. In addition, humidity was measured by various measuring methods so that a comparison of the published results is difficult.

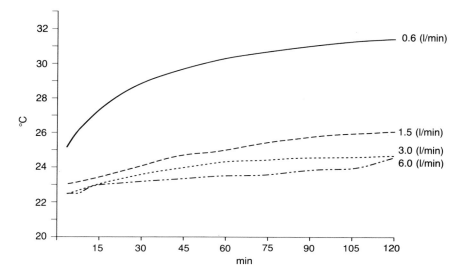

Figure 6.8 Temperature of anaesthetic gas at different fresh gas flows during 2 h of anaesthesia (From Kleemann[35], by permission)

6.4.1 Breathing gas temperature

Kleemann[34,35] showed that after 2 h of anaesthesia with a fresh gas flow of 0.6 l/min, the inspired breathing gas temperature had increased to an average of 31.5°C. Although this high value is only achieved after about 90 min, the gas temperature rises to about 28°C within the first 30 min. The temperatures measured during low flow anaesthesia were at all times distinctly higher than those measured with a high fresh gas flow (Figure 6.8). Buijs points out that the high breathing gas temperature of 36–40°C which is measured directly downstream of the carbon dioxide absorber with low flow anaesthesia is rapidly reduced to 20–24°C by heat losses in the inspired limb of the patient hose system[14]. And yet, using a circle rebreathing system with a fresh gas flow of 0.5 l/min, Bengtson measured gas temperatures of 28.5°C, which were about 6.8°C above room temperature after a period of 30 min. These temperatures were higher than those measured with non-rebreathing systems, even though these were additionally equipped with passive heat and moisture exchangers (artificial noses)[32]. In another comparative examination with absorber canisters of 4.7 and 0.9 litre volume, Bengtson comes to the conclusion that the breathing gas temperature with low flow anaesthesia is favourably influenced by absorber canisters of comparatively small volumes[36].

6.4.2 Breathing gas humidity

If anaesthesia is performed with a rebreathing system using low fresh gas flow, the humidity is likewise higher than with high fresh gas flows. Following

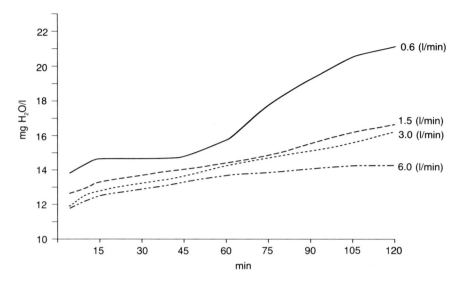

Figure 6.9 Humidity of anaesthetic gas at different fresh gas flows during 2 h of anaesthesia (From Kleemann[35], by permission)

2 h anaesthesia with a fresh gas flow of 0.6 l/min, Kleemann found an average inspired humidity of 21 mg H_2O/l in the breathing gases. However, it takes a certain latency period (Figure 6.9) for the humidity in the breathing gas to rise to sufficient values, comparable to the rise in temperature of the breathing gases. While Kleemann established 60–75 min for this latency period in his measurements, this period amounts to just 30 min according to Bengtson's investigations. He measured an absolute humidity of 28 mg H_2O/l in the breathing gases after 60 min with a fresh gas flow of 0.5 l/min[32,36]. The humidity values measured in the breathing gas after completion of the equilibrium period again correspond approximately to the values established if passive heat and moisture exchangers are used.

6.4.3   Body temperature

Improved climatization of anaesthetic gases reduces the heat and fluid losses which occur in the respiratory tract when dry gas is warmed up and humidified by the epithelium. The effect is to reduce the decrease in body temperature that is usually observed[37-39]. There is just one clinical study available which confirms that the body temperature can be maintained merely by reduction of the fresh gas flow when closed system anaesthesia is performed[40], After an initial average temperature drop of 0.8°C during the first 60 min, the body temperature rises within the next hour to the starting value established at the beginning of anaesthesia (Figure 6.10). However, in performing closed system anaesthesia, Buijs demonstrated a persistant drop of 1.6°C in oesophageal temperature within 120 min[14]. It must be remembered though that the heat losses with respiration amount to about 15 kcal/h for

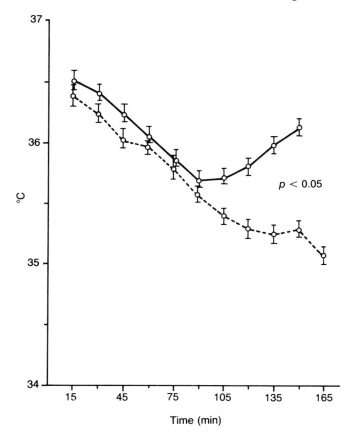

Figure 6.10   Average oesophageal temperature: (———) closed system anaesthesia; (————)
anaesthesia with semi-closed rebreathing system using 5 l/min fresh gas flow (From Aldrete[40],
by permission)

an uncovered narcotized patient, being only around 10% of the total net
loss of energy amounting to about 150 kcal/h. Although the net heat loss
can be reduced to 30 kcal/h if the narcotized patient is well protected by
covers or is wrapped in reflective blankets, there remains 50% of heat losses
which are unaffected by variation of the fresh gas flow.

6.4.4   Implications for anaesthetic practice

The following statements seem to be justified concerning improvement of
anaesthetic gas climatization by reduction of the fresh gas flow:

1. Temperature and humidity of anaesthetic gases increase if rebreathing
   systems are used with low fresh gas flow leading the already warm and
   moist exhaled gas back to the patient.

2. If minimal flow anaesthesia is performed with a fresh gas flow of 0.5 l/min, the values of anaesthetic gas temperature and humidity attained after an equilibrium period of 60 min come very close to values between 28°C and 32°C and 17–30 mgH$_2$O/l, which are considered as being nearly optimal. They correspond approximately to those values, which can be gained by the use of passive heat and moisture exchangers.
3. The protection of morphological integrity[34] and function[36] of the tracheobronchial ciliated epithelium, as a result of improved breathing gas climatization by flow reduction, can be impressively verified by animal experiments and clinical examination.
4. Warming and humidification of breathing gases can be considerably improved if the fresh gas is routed through an absorber whose volume is not too great (about 1 litre), and heat losses are kept low by appropriate choice of materials and dimensions of the patient hose system.
5. Adequate climatization of the breathing gas is a valuable contribution with respect to maintaining the body temperature of a narcotized patient[40,41].
6. The advantages of improving the anaesthetic gas climate by anaesthesia management with low fresh gas flow will be most marked in prolonged anaesthetics.

6.5   Extended potentials of patient monitoring and improved knowledge of machine functions

The monitoring potentials inherent in the utilization of rebreething systems cannot be quantitatively assessed in the same manner as their aforementioned advantages. With regard to anaesthesia management with reduced fresh gas flow, it is an advantage in itself, however, to deal with the characteristics and function of breathing systems, the technical concepts of anaesthetic machines, and the regularities involved in the uptake and distribution of oxygen, nitrous oxide and volatile anaesthetics. In addition, the reduction of fresh gas flow calls for careful equipment maintenance which is itself beneficial for patients. A commitment to closed system anaesthesia and anaesthesia management with low fresh gas flows discloses new perspectives to the anaesthetist, leading to a better understanding of both patient and anaesthetic machine[13,42,43].

If available technical equipment permits the performance of quantitative closed system anaesthesia, it will enable precise determination and continuous monitoring of oxygen consumption, uptake of volatile anaesthetics and carbon dioxide production, which in turn facilitates comprehensive evaluation of metabolic, respiratory and circulatory conditions[12,44–48].

6.6   References

1. Feiss, P., Demontoux, M. H. and Colin, D. Anesthetic gas and vapour saving with minimal flow anesthesia. *Acta Anesth. Belg.*, **41**, 249–251 (1990)

2. Pedersen, F. M., Nielsen, J., Ibsen, M. and Guldager, H. Low-flow isoflurane–nitrous oxide anaesthesia offers substantial economic advantages over high-flow and medium flow isoflurane–nitrous oxide anaesthesia. *Acta Anaesth. Scand.*, **37**, 509–512 (1993)

3. Cotter, S. M., Petros, A. J., Dor, C. J., Berber, N. D. and White, D. C. Low-flow anaesthesia. *Anaesthesia*, **46**, 1009–1012 (1991)

4. Baum, J. A. and Aitkenhead, A. R. Low flow anaesthesia. *Anaesthesia*, **50** (Suppl.), 37–44 (1995)

5. Baum, J. Die Narkose mit niedrigem Frischgasfluß: Darstellung des Verfahrens in Frage und Antwort. Bibliomed, Med. Verl. Ges., Melsungen (1993)

6. Loke, J. and Shearer, W. A. J. Cost of anaesthesia. *Can. J. Anaesth.*, **40**, 472–474 (1993)

7. Droh, R. and Rothmann, G. Das geschlossene Kreisystem. *Anaesthesist*, **26**, 461–466 (1977)

8. Ernst, E. A. and Spain, J. A. Closed-circuit and high-flow systems: examining alternatives. In *Future Anesthesia Delivery Systems* (ed. B. R. Brown), *Contemporary Anesthesia Practice*, Vol. 8, F. A. Davies, Philadelphia (1984), pp. 11–38

9. Matjasko, J. Economic impact of low-flow anaesthesia. *Anesthesiology*, **67**, 863–864 (1987)

10. Herscher, E. and Yeakel, A. E. Nitrous oxide–oxygen based anesthesia: the waste and its cost. *Anaesth. Rev.*, **4**, 29 (1977)

11. Bengtson, J. P., Sonander, H. and Stenqvist, O. Comparison of costs of different anaesthetic techniques. *Acta Anaesthesiol. Scand.*, **32**, 33–35 (1988)

12. Christensen, K. N., Thomsen, A., Jorgensen, S. and Fabricius, J. Analysis of costs of anaesthetic breathing systems. *Br. J. Anaesth.*, **59**, 389–390 (1987)

13. Edsall, D. W. Economy is not a major benefit of closed-system anesthesia. *Anesthesiology*, **54**, 258–259 (1981)

14. Buijs, B. H. M. J. Herwardering van het Gesloten Ademsysteem in de Anesthesiologie. Dissertationsschrift der Erasmus-Universität, Rotterdam (1988)

15. Baum, J., Enzenauer, J., Krausse, Th. and Sachs, G. Atemkalk-Nutzungsdauer, Verbrauch und Kosten in Abhängigkeit vom Frischgasfluß. *Anaesthesiol. Reanimat.*, **18**, 108–113 (1993)

16. Pothmann, W., Shimada, K., Goerig, M. and Fuhlrott, M. J. Schulte am Esch: Belastungen des Arbeitsplatzes durch Naroksegase. *Anaesthesist*, **40**, 339–346 (1991)

17. Spence, A. A. Environmental pollution by inhalation anaesthetics. *Br. J. Anaesth.*, **59**, 96–103 (1987)

18. Waterson, C. K. Recovery of waste anesthetic gases. In *Future Anesthesia Delivery Systems* (ed. B. R. Brown), *Contemporary Anesthesia Practice*, Vol. VIII, Davis, Philadelphia (1984), pp. 109–124

19. Deutsche Forschungsgemeinschaft. Maximale Arbeitsplatzkonzentrationen und biologische Arbeitsstofftoleranzwerte (1994).

20. Amt Für Arbeitsschutz: Merkblatt für den Umgang mit Narkosegasen, Stand August 1990. Freie und Hansestadt Hamburg, Behörde für Arbeit, Gesundheit and Soziales, Hamburg (1990)

21. Virtue, R. W. Low flow anesthesia: advantages in its clinical application, cost and ecology. In *Low Flow and Closed System Anesthesia* (eds J. A. Aldrete, H. J. Lowe and R. W. Virtue), Grune and Stratton, New York (1979), pp. 103–108

22. Logan, M. and Farmer, J. G. Anaesthesia and the ozone layer. *Br. J. Anaesth.*, **53**, 645–646 (1989)

23. Graul, E. H. and Forth, W. Das 'gute' Ozon. *Dt. Ärztebl.*, **87**, 2284–2291 (1990)

24. Sherman, S. J. and Cullen, B. F. Nitrous oxide and the greenhouse effect. *Anesthesiology*, **68** 816–817 (1988)

25. Hoechst. Umweltwirkung der Fluor-Chlor-Kohlenwassertoffe (FCKW) und ihre Bedeutung für die Anästhesie. Stellungnahme der Fa. Hoechst, Frankfurt a. M., vom 04.09.1989

26. Hutton, P. and Kerr, J. A. Anaesthetic agents and the ozone layer. *Lancet*, 1011 (1989)

27. Pierce, J. M. T. and Linter, S. P. K. Anaesthetic agents and the ozone layer. *Lancet*, 1011–1012 (1989)

28. Radke, J. and Fabian, P. Die Ozonschicht und ihre Beeinflussung durch N_2O und Inhalationsanästhetika. *Anaesthesist*, **40**, 429–433 (1991)

29. Noerreslet, J., Frieberg, S., Nielsen, T. M. and Römer, U. Halothane anaesthetic and the ozone layer. *Lancet*, 719 (1989)
30. Aldrete, J. A., Cubillos, P. and Sherrill, D. Humidity and temperature changes during low flow and closed system anaesthesia. *Acta Anaesth. Scand.*, **25**, 312–314 (1981)
31. Wick, C., Altemeyer, K. H., Ahnefeld, F. W. and Kilian, J. Vergleichende Feuchtigkeits-messungen in halbgeschlossenen und halboffenen Systemen unter zusätzlicher Verwendung von Künstlichen Nasen. *Anaesthesist*, **36**, 172–176 (1987)
32. Bengtson, J. P., Sonander, H. and Stenqvist, O. Preservation of humidity and heat of respiratory gases during anaesthesia – a laboratory investigation. *Acta Anaesthesiol. Scand.*, **31**, 127–131 (1987)
33. Chalon, J., Ali, M., Turndorf, H. and Fischgrund, G. K. *Humidification of Anesthetic Gases*, Charles C. Thomas, Springfield, Ill. (1981)
34. Kleemann, P. P. Tierexperimentelle und klinische Untersuchungen zum Stellenwert der Klimatisierung anästhetischer Gase im Narkosekreissystem bei Langzeiteingriffen. Wissen-schaftliche Verlagsabteilung Abbott GmbH, Wiesbaden (1989)
35. Kleemann, P. P. Klimatisierung anästhetischer Gase durch Reduktion des Frischgasflows. In *Narkosebeatmung – Low Flow, Minimal Flow, Geschlossens System* (eds J.-P. A. H. Jantzen and P. P. Kleemann), Schattauer, Stuttgart 1989, pp. 101–123
36. Bengtson, J. P., Bengtson, A. and Stenqvist, O. The circle system as a humidifier. *Br. J. Anaesth.*, **63**, 453–457 (1989)
37. Imrie, M. M. and Hall, G. M. Body temperature and anaesthesia. *Br. J. Anaesth.*, **64**, 346–354 (1990)
38. Newton, D. E. F. The effect of anaesthetic gas humidification on body temperature. *Br. J. Anaesth.*, **47**, 1026 (1975)
39. Stone, D. R., Downs, J. B., Paul, W. L. and Perkins, H. M. Adult body temperature and heated humidification of anesthetic gases during general anesthesia. *Anesth. Analg.*, **60**, 736–741 (1981)
40. Aldrete, J. A. Closed circuit anesthesia prevents moderate hypothermia occurring in patients having extremity surgery. *Circular*, **4**, 3–4 (1987)
41. Scherer, R., Brendle, B. C. and Lawin, P. Minimal-Flow-Anästhesie und vorgewärmte Infusionslösungen zur Vermeidung von intraoperativer Hypothermie bei Wirbelsäulen-operationen. *Anästh. Intensivmed.*, **28**, 249–252 (1987)
42. Baum, J. Quantitative anaesthesia in the low-flow system. In *Quantitative Anaesthesia: Low Flow and Closed Circuit* (eds K. H. Frankenberger, E. Konecny and K. Steinbereithner), *Anaesthesiology and Intensive Care Medicine*, Vol. 204, Springer, Berlin (1989), pp. 44–57
43. Cullen, S. C. Who is watching the patient? *Anesthesiology*, **37**, 361–362 (1972)
44. Spieß, W. Narkose im geschlossenen System mit kontinuierlicher inspiratorischer Sauer-stoffmessung. *Anaesthesist*, **26**, 503–513 (1977)
45. Van der Zee, H. and Verkaaik, A. P. K. Cardiovascular implementations of respiratory measurements. *Acta Anaesth. Belg.*, **41**, 167–175 (1990)
46. Verkaaik, A. P. K. and Erdmann, W. Respiratory diagnostic possibilities during closed circuit anesthesia. *Acta Anaesth. Belg.*, **41**, 177–188 (1990)
47. Versichelen, L. and Rolly, G. Mass-spectrometric evaluation of some recently introduced low flow, closed circuit systems. *Acta Anaesth. Belg.*, **41**, 225–237 (1990)
48. Westenskow, D. R. and Loughlin, P. J. Quantitative anaesthesia with the help of closed-loop control. In *Quantitative Anaesthesia: Low Flow and Closed Circuit* (eds K. Van Ackern, H. Frankenberger, E. Konecny and K. Steinbereithner), *Anaesthesiology and Intensive Care Medicine*, Vol. 204, Springer, Berlin (1989), pp. 109–119

Technical requirements for anaesthesia management with reduced fresh gas flow

7.1 Technical regulations and standards

In several countries there are already binding national regulations concerning technical features and mandatory safety devices for inhalational anaesthetic machines, the negligence of which may be subject to medicolegal consequences in the event of any complication.

In the German-speaking countries, regulations concerning the technical properties of anaesthetic machines are in force: DIN 13 252 in Germany, ÖNORM K2003 in Austria and SN 057 600 in Switzerland. A common European Standard, prEN 740 'Anaesthetic Workstations and their Modules – Essential Requirements', is submitted for formal vote and will be binding for all manufacturers and anaesthetists in the countries of the European Community[1]. In Germany, newly built anaesthetic machines which have been put into operation since June 1991 already have to comply with the technical requirements given by the draft of the DIN 13 252 A1[2] which are nearly identical to the outline of the new European standard. In January 1993 the draft of the International Standard on Anaesthetic Machines for Use with Humans, ISO 5358 2nd edn was presented[3]. In the USA, Standard Specifications for anaesthetic ventilators (ASTM designation: F 1101-90), for components and systems of anaesthetic gas machines (ASTM designation F 1161-88), and for anaesthesia breathing systems (ASTM designation F 1208-89) are available[4].

Furthermore, if performing low flow anaesthesia, the anaesthesist should be aware whether this anaesthetic technique is covered by the specification of the particular anaesthetic machine in use.

7.2 Technical requirements for the anaesthetic equipment with respect to the extent of fresh gas flow reduction

7.2.1 Medical gas supply systems

All three variants of anaesthesia management with reduced fresh gas flow place no special technical requirements on the gas supply system. A nitrous oxide cut-off and an audible oxygen failure signal are mandatory technical safety facilities for inhalational anaesthetic machines under prEN 740.

7.2.2   Flow control systems

Nitrous oxide and oxygen are either controlled individually at the respective flow control system or as premixed gas, having passed a calibrated blender. In the majority of machines, the gas flow is adjusted at fine needle valves and measured with conventional flowmeter tubes. Alternatively, the gas flow can be measured electronically and may be displayed either numerically or by an analogue scale. The requirements placed on the valve function and the calibration and graduation of gas flow control systems increase in line with the degree of flow reduction[5,6].

Low flow anaesthesia can be performed with flow control systems of all common types of anaesthetic machines. Even where older machines are concerned, the nitrous oxide and oxygen flow can be accurately set to at least 500 ml/min at the controls.

Performance of minimal flow anaesthesia calls for more precisely calibrated flowmeter tubes which, starting with a gas flow of 50–100 ml/min, must be graduated in increments of 50 ml/min, but at least 100 ml/min. This requirement is satisfied by the new generation of anaesthetic machines, the majority of which are equipped with double flowmeter tubes for exact control of oxygen and nitrous oxide even over the lowest flow range.

The accuracy of gas measurement readings in the low flow range is quoted as being 10% by the different standards[1–4,7]. For performance of minimal flow anaesthesia, which is by no means a quantitative method, this error is acceptable for use in clinical routine. A tolerance of 10% deviation between real gas flow and displayed value may even be acceptable as an international technical standard[8].

In this context, the reader's attention is drawn to an incident observed by the author. Using a brand new anaesthetic machine it was noticed that, after about 15 minutes of anaesthesia, the float in the flowmeter tube no longer moved freely. The rotating movement of the float ceased, it then dropped down in the unchanged gas flow, and it was clear that it was partially tilted and jammed in the metering tube. On checking these flowmeter tubes, we noticed that in this case of malfunction the oxygen volume supplied was 100–150 ml/min higher than that indicated by the bobbin. Inaccuracies in calibration of the flowmeter tubes up to 50% max. have also been described by Saunders et al.[9]. On the other hand, the precision of flowmeter tubes was adjudged satisfactory by Rügheimer[10]. It could be demonstrated later, that this malfunction, which could be observed in all anaesthetic machines of this series, was attributable to a manufacturing fault.

In dealing with this case of malfunction, a fundamental problem deserves emphasis. Since most are accustomed to using high excess gas volumes, routine technical maintenance and checks to verify that the flow control systems conform to the tolerances in the low flow range specified by the manufacturer are often neglected. It is important that, prior to performance of low flow anaesthesia, the flow control systems should be carefully tested for accurate function especially in the low flow range.

Closed system anaesthesia can only be realized provided that the anaesthetic machine is fitted with flow control systems which, starting with 50 ml/min, are graduated in increments of 10 ml over the low flow range. This is the only way to ensure that gas volumes which correspond to the actual oxygen and nitrous oxide uptake of the patient can be appropriately adjusted at the machine. Fine flow tubes with such accurate graduation are available for instance as an option for the Cicero anaesthetic machine (Drägerwerk, Lübeck, Germany) (Figure 7.1).

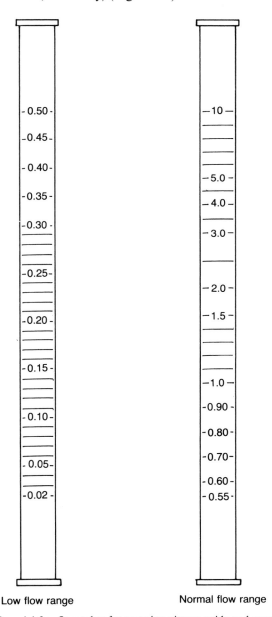

Low flow range   Normal flow range

Figure 7.1   Set of special fine flow tubes for metering nitrous oxide and oxygen; the graduation in the low flow range permits reduction down to closed system anaesthesia flows (From Frankenberger[11], by permission)

With such low gas flows, however, the imprecise performance of needle valves presents a problem[7]. The repeated correction of oxygen and nitrous oxide settings takes a lot of time and attention on the part of the anaesthetist. Furthermore, the Oxygen Ratio Monitor Controller (ORMC) (North American Dräger, Telford, Pennsylvania, USA), with its pneumatic coupling of the oxygen to the nitrous oxide flow, makes it exceptionally difficult to adjust very small gas flows exactly[12].

Special problems also result from fresh gas control by a gas mixer, as is the case for example in the AV 1 anaesthetic machine (Drägerwerk, Lübeck, Germany). Once oxygen and nitrous oxide have been mixed in the desired ratio, the flow of mixed gas has to be adjusted at a flowmeter calibrated for a defined gas mixture (consisting of 40% O_2 and 60% N_2O). However, the density of the mixed gas is reduced with increasing oxygen portion, so that the resultant gas flow is actually higher than that indicated by the flowmeter. Although this fault can be tolerated in low flow and minimal flow anaesthesia, the accuracy of the mixed-gas flowmeter tube does not satisfy the requirements for quantitative closed system anaesthesia. However, as the calibration of the AV 1 mixed-gas flowmeter tube starts only at a minimum flow of 400 ml/min, this machine cannot be used with flows less than 500 ml/min. The same applies for instance to the Siemens Anesthesia System: once the fresh gas has passed the blender, it is not possible to select a flow less than 500 ml/min with the required accuracy[13].

The precision of gas blending, which is quoted for the Dräger gas mixer as being $\pm 4\%$ with arbitrary nitrous oxide–oxygen mixtures, and for the Siemens Elema blender with $\pm 5\%$, is suitable for performance of low flow and minimal flow anaesthesia in routine clinical practice.

7.2.3   Vaporizers

7.2.3.1   Precision

It is general practice today that volatile anaesthetics are admixed to the fresh gas, i.e. the vaporizers are connected into the fresh gas supply (VOC, vaporizer outside the circle). For performance of low flow anaesthesia, use should be made of precision plenum vaporizers. In addition to pressure and temperature compensation, they should deliver the preset concentration reliably even with very low fresh gas flows. In conventional plenum vaporizers this is guaranteed by their laminar flow characteristics[14]. The high flow constancy of Vapor 19.n vaporizers (Drägerwerk, Lübeck, Germany) (Figure 7.2), was confirmed by Züchner[16] and Gilly[17], even for extremely low gas flows down to 20 ml/min. The performance characteristics concerning flow constancy of the TEC 5 (Ohmeda, Hatfield, UK) or the Penlon PPV sigma (Penlon, Abingdon, UK) vaporizers are also adequate for performance of low flow anaesthesia[18]. But if older type vaporizers are still used, such as the TEC 2, the anaesthetist has to expect pronounced flow dependency. This adverse performance characteristic may be augmented under controlled ventilation, as the vaporizer additionally is subject to a distinct pumping effect[19].

The precision of the concentration supplied is also a function of the fresh gas composition; this dependency decreases with a reduction of flow and an increase of the set concentration.

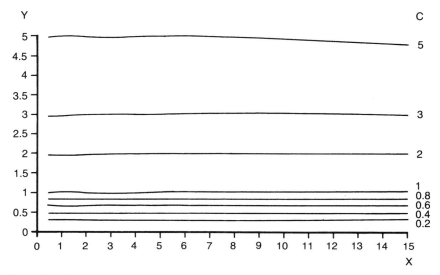

Figure 7.2 Flow constancy of the Vapor 19.n vaporizer (Drägerwerk, Lübeck, Germany): precise performance over a flow range of 0.4–15 l/min (C, concentration set on isoflurane vaporizer, vol%; X, fresh gas flow rate; Y, isoflurane fresh gas concentration, vol%)[15]

The so-called 'pumping effect' (effect of pressure change during controlled ventilation) on the concentration supplied by the vaporizer can be reduced by taking care that the vaporizer chamber is always adequately filled if low concentrations are set during anaesthesia with low flow[14].

In summarizing the results of his investigations, Gilly[17] points out that the concentration supplied even from modern plenum vaporizers may vary greatly as a function of flow and composition of the carrier gas. The nominal and delivered value of anaesthetic agent concentration will differ by up to 20% if several parameters are varied simultaneously. These vaporizers are nevertheless suitable for use with low flow anaesthesia. Differences between the anaesthetic concentrations set at the vaporizer and that actually supplied are buffered by the gas volume of the breathing system which is large in relation to the fresh gas volume. Furthermore, changes in anaesthetic gas composition occur very slowly with low flow anaesthesia because of the particularly long time constant. If the requirements imposed on the precision of vaporizer performance are solely evaluated in terms of patient safety, however, with decreasing fresh gas flow the specification need not be so demanding.

However, quantitative closed system anaesthesia cannot be performed with conventional plenum vaporizers. Their inadequate precision neither allows exact metering and supply of defined anaesthetic volumes, nor a sufficiently accurate determination of the amount of anaesthetic being taken up by the patient.

The vaporizer's dependency on gas composition and flow can be reduced with the aid of an alternative technical concept in which the anaesthetic is fed into the fresh gas flow as defined quanta. The Gambro-Engström anaesthetic delivery systems employ this principle[20,21]. In the Elsa,

EAS 9010 and EAS 9020 anaesthetic machines (Gambro-Engström, Bromma, Sweden), the liquid anaesthetic is injected under pressure into a heated vaporizer chamber. The anaesthetic vapour is then admixed to the fresh gas in defined boluses via an electronically controlled pulsating valve whose frequency is related directly to the fresh gas flow (Figure 7.3).

The performance of the Servo Anaesthesia System's vaporizer (Siemens-Elema, Solna, Sweden) is also flow independent[13]: the liquid agent is sprayed by gas pressure via a nozzle directly into a fresh gas stream of intermittent flow (Figure 7.4). Corresponding to its calibration to 400 or 350 kPa (= 4 or

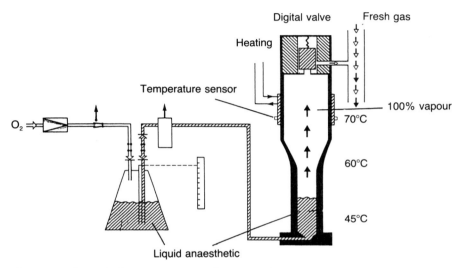

Figure 7.3 Electronically controlled device for supply of anaesthetic vapour in defined boluses (Gambro-Engström, Bromma, Sweden) (From Frankenberger[22], by permission)

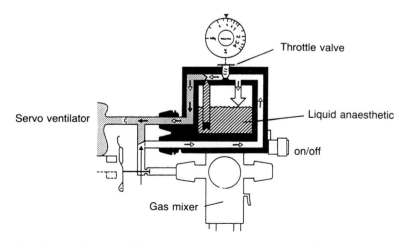

Figure 7.4 Siemens Vaporizer 950; the liquid anaesthetic agent is sprayed by gas pressure via a nozzle directly into the fresh gas stream

3.5 bar), the exact performance of this type of vaporizer essentially depends on the precise control of the gas pressure at 450 ± 30 kPa or 360 ± 30 kPa, respectively. If the central piped medical gas is supplied with a higher pressure of about 520 to 550 kPa, unexpected high concentrations, 60–100% higher than the dial setting, may be delivered by this vaporizer. In this case, the use of an additional pressure regulator switched into the pipeline connections to the gas mixer is indispensable[23].

However, Gilly remarks critically on this subject that, although the amount of anaesthetic supplied to the fresh gas may be more accurately metered with such improved dosing systems, the inaccuracies of the flow control systems counteract the precision potentially offered by these devices[17].

7.2.3.2 Limitation of vaporizer output

Anaesthesia management with low fresh gas flow is rendered difficult in so far as the output of nearly all vaporizers is limited to a value of about $3 \times$ MAC (minimal alveolar concentration), commonly in halothane vaporizers to 4% or 5%, in those for enflurane and isoflurane to 5% in sevoflurane vaporizers to 8%, and in desflurane vaporizers to 18%. The maximum output of these vaporizers decreases furthermore in direct proportion to the extent of fresh gas flow reduction. The difficulty mentioned applies to all situations in which a comparatively large amount of anaesthetic vapour is to be added into the breathing system when simultaneously the fresh gas flow is to be kept low, for instance during the induction phase with its wash-in processes and initial high uptake or during the course of anaesthesia, if the anaesthetic depth is to be increased within a short period of time. If the demand for anaesthetic vapour is high, the limited amount being supplied by an output-limited vaporizer with low fresh gas flow may be too low. Even though the vaporizer may be set to its maximum output of up to 5%, the anaesthetic vapour which is fed into the system will not amount to more than 25 ml/min at a gas flow of 0.5 l/min.

The anaesthetic concentration can only be rapidly increased in spite of a low fresh gas flow, if the following procedures and technical alternatives are adopted:

- demand-specific supply of the anaesthetic agents by direct injection of the liquid anaesthetic into the breathing system
- use of precise injection systems independent of the fresh gas flow[11]
- use of vaporizers which are switched into the breathing system (VIC, vaporizer inside the circle) so that the anaesthetic can be supplied without being influenced in any way by the adjustment of the fresh gas flow, or
- increase of the output limits of vaporizers which are connected into the fresh gas flow (VOC).

Intermittent manual injection of the volatile anaesthetic into the system will not be recommended for clinical practice, as has already been pointed out. It is extremely involved, especially during the initial phase of anaesthesia, and whenever rapid changes in the agent's concentration are required. Switching the vaporizer into the breathing system must be rejected with a view to patient's safety, particularly in the case of controlled ventilation, since dangerously high anaesthetic concentrations may be rapidly achieved, especially in flow anaesthesia, unless stringent monitoring standards are met. At present, the only machines which are equipped with precisely operating injection dosage systems are Elsa, EAS 9010 and EAS 9020 (Gambro-Engström, Bromma, Sweden) and PhysioFlex (Physio B.V., Haarlem, The Netherlands). According to investigations by Versichelen and Rolly, these dosage devices work accurately and reliably in clinical use[24]. The use of vaporizers with increased output limits would be a simple and practicable alternative. Since changes in anaesthetic gas concentration proceed very slowly in low flow anaesthesia, even though the anaesthetic concentration in the fresh gas may have been drastically changed, the use of such a vaporizer would not present an increased risk for the patient. An additional safeguard against accidental overdose would be a mechanical device which needs to be unlocked before the vaporizer concentration exceeds 5%. However, conventional plenum vaporizers with increased output are not available for use in human medicine, for safety reasons and due to various national regulations, e.g. DIN13252[25]. The Elsa is the only machine in which the output of the dosage system has been increased to 8%, for halothane, enflurane and for isoflurane likewise.

At present, anaesthetists have to change to high fresh gas flows whenever a large volume of anaesthetic vapour has to be supplied into the system rapidly by a conventional vaporizer.

7.2.3.3 Specified range of operation

The operation range specified by the manufacturer for reasons of liability may be an impediment to the user and, sometimes, seems to be substantially unjustified. For instance, in accordance with its Instructions for Use, the Vapor 19.1 (Drägerwerk, Lübeck, Germany)[15] is approved for use in anaesthesia with rebreathing and non-rebreathing systems. The flow range is quoted as being between 0.3 and 15 l/min. However, according to the Instructions for Use (April 1986), the usage range of the Vapor 19.n is restricted as follows: 'The Vapor is approved for use with semi-closed and semi-open systems, but should not be used with closed, or nearly closed breathing systems', leaving unexplained, what is meant by the term 'nearly closed'. The arbitrary establishment of the vaporizer's lower flow range limit to 0.5 l/min seems especially unfounded if they are attached to machines which are equipped with the optionally available fine flow tubes. This fact has been considered in the latest version of the Instructions for Use, dated March 1991, where the lower limit of the vaporizer's operation range is again quoted as being 250 ml/min, so that its use with even lower flows is not definitively precluded.

7.2.3.4 The Tec 6 desflurane vaporizer

The pharmacokinetic properties of desflurane justify the expectation that this agent will be especially suitable for low flow anaesthesia; thus a short paragraph is devoted to the Tec 6 vaporizer (Ohmeda, Steeton, UK)[26,27]. Due to the high vapour pressure of desflurane at room temperature, the desflurane (Tec 6) vaporizer is, unlike the other conventional plenum vaporizers, an electronically controlled device. The fluid desflurane is heated to 39°C, thus providing a constant vapour pressure of 1460 mmHg. An electronically controlled regulator delivers just that amount of vaporized desflurane which, mixed with the carrier gas flow, results in the preset fresh gas concentration. Several safety features are incorporated into this device. A shut-off valve only opens the connection between the vaporizing chamber and the regulator if the device is operational, electrically powered and placed correctly on the back bar of the anaesthetic machine. In case of angular displacement exceeding 15° from the vertical position, a 'tilt switch' activates the shut-off valve, thus preventing liquid desflurane from leaving the sump. 0.2 to 10 l/min are the specified working limits of the desflurane vaporizer. Using pure oxygen as carrier gas at a flow between 5 and 10 l/min, the desflurane concentration in the outflow gas is within 15% relative or 0.5% absolute of the dial setting, as specified. At flow rates less than 2 l/min, the desflurane concentration is generally about 8% smaller than at larger carrier gas flow rates, but is still within the above limits. If the dialled concentration exceeds 12%, in the fresh gas flow range less than 1 l/min the output concentration can be up to 1% higher than the dial setting. Due to the lower viscosity, with 70% nitrous oxide in oxygen the output concentration can be 20% less than the dial setting[26,28]. The output performance of the Tec 6 desflurane vaporizer, as specified, satisfies the requirements for safe performance of low and minimal flow anaesthesia.

7.2.4 Breathing systems

For rebreathing techniques, use can basically be made of both the to-and-fro and the circle absorption system. To-and-fro absorption systems are rarely used today since working with absorber canisters mounted near the patient is awkward and carbon dioxide absorption may become insufficient with increasing duration of anaesthesia[29]. Circle systems can be used in all different techniques of anaesthesia with low fresh gas flow. However, the technical demands placed on the rebreathing systems increase with decreasing fresh gas flow.

7.2.4.1 Gas tightness

Virtually all anaesthetic machines should be suitable for anaesthesia with a fresh gas flow of 1 l/min, assuming they are well maintained. It is necessary, however, to check the breathing systems for leaks in accordance with the manufacturer's instructions to ensure that quoted leakage tolerances are not exceeded. Under these provisions, low flow anaesthesia can be undertaken without any further technical effort.

The requirements concerning the gas tightness of the systems are higher in minimal flow anaesthesia. With a pressure of 2 kPa ($\simeq 20\,cmH_2O$) within the system, gas loss resulting from leaks should not exceed 100 ml/min. The required gas tightness can be achieved by careful cleaning of rubber seals and replacement if they are brittle, as well as careful tightening of screw connections in the circle system. Plastic components must be checked for brittleness and cracks, and have to be replaced if required. In addition, attention must be paid to the proper mounting of carefully cleaned taper connections (Figure 7.5).

Manufacturers quote the following leakage tolerances for their respective

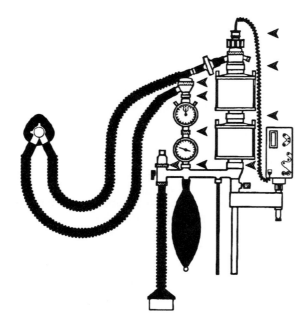

Figure 7.5   Points predisposed to leaks demonstrated on a conventional circle absorber system 8 ISO (Drägerwerk, Lübeck, Germany): all screw and plug connections and the valve and absorber seals.

breathing systems. The leakage rate of the 8 ISO breathing system (Drägerwerk, Lübeck, Germany) must not exceed 200 ml/min at an internal system pressure of 4 kPa ($\simeq 40$ cmH$_2$O)[15]; a leak rate of less than 50 ml/min is quoted for the Megamed 048 and 219 circle systems (Megamed, Cham, Switzerland) at a pressure of 3 kPa ($\simeq 30$ cmH$_2$O)[30]. The automatic leak test performed on the Cicero anaesthetic workstation (Drägerwerk, Lübeck, Germany) at 3 kPa ($\simeq 30$ cmH$_2$O)[15] results, according to the author's experience, in average values between 20 and 40 ml/min. An automatic leak test at 3 kPa ($\simeq 30$ cmH$_2$O) is also carried out by the Elsa, the EAS 9010 and the EAS 9020 anaesthetic machines (Gambro Engström, Bromma, Sweden)[20]. The compact circle absorber system of the Ohmeda CD anaesthetic machine (Ohmeda, Hatfield, UK) also proved to be highly gas tight. With the Servo Anaesthesia Circle System 985 (Siemens-Elema, Solna, Sweden) the leak test of the breathing system and identification of leaks is quite difficult as the test cannot be performed under static conditions but only during operation of the ventilator. The author's own experiences confirm the results of investigations concerning gas leakage of breathing systems published by Leuenberger[31]. All circle absorber systems tested performed below the leakage limit of 100 ml/min at a pressure of 3 kPa ($\simeq 30$ cmH$_2$O) as proposed by the draft of the Common European Standard[1]. The Authority for Occupational Safety and Health, Hamburg, provides in its Instruction Sheet on the Handling of Anaesthetic Gases that the breathing system should be checked for leaks at a pressure of 3 kPa ($\simeq 30$ cmH$_2$O) several times per day, and that leaks in excess of 100 ml/min should not be accepted[32]. All breathing systems which indicate such low leakage loss satisfy the technical requirements placed on gas tightness for performance of anaesthesia even with the lowest fresh gas flows.

Performance of closed system anaesthesia requires a rebreathing system to be leakproof to the greatest possible extent. The connections between the individual components of the system, and tapers in particular, must fit each other perfectly and be coated with a sealing paste (e.g. Oxygenox S4, Drägerwerk, Lübeck, Germany). The number of connections should be restricted to a minimum. It is proven practice to mark all individual components of a gas tight circle system and to fit the appropriate components of the same circle system together for reassembly[33]. On the other hand, the compact breathing systems of the new generation machines (Cato, Cicero, EAS 9010 and 9020, Elsa, Megamed 700, Modulus) are in general so gas tight that, without further prerequisites, they cope with the requirements for closed system anaesthesia, assuming appropriate maintenance[24,34].

7.2.4.2 Fresh gas utilization

Utilization of fresh gas will be explained by the example of the 8 ISO circle absorption system (Drägerwerk, Lübeck, Germany). The degree of fresh gas utilization increases with increasing reduction of the fresh gas flow and reaches about 100% in the minimal flow range. With a higher fresh gas flow this value amounts to only about 70% (Figure 7.6). Fresh gas utilization is also determined by the design of the system that is, by the position of the fresh gas inlet in relation to the excess gas discharge valve, as well as by its flow characteristics[35,36] (Figure 7.7). In the case of the AV 1 (Drägerwerk, Lübeck, Germany), fresh gas utilization is optimized by a rebreathing gas exchanger (see Figure 7.15b), while in the Cicero (Drägerwerk, Lübeck, Germany) utilization is optimized by the position of the fresh gas supply

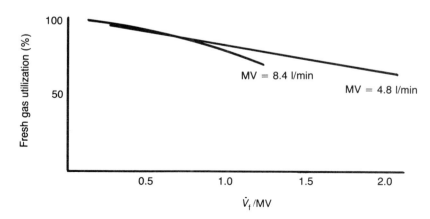

Figure 7.6 Fresh gas utilization of a conventional circle absorber system 8 ISO (Drägerwerk, Lübeck, Germany), illustrated as a function of quotient of fresh gas flow ($\dot{V}_f$) and minute volume (MV) (From von dem Hagen and Kleinschmidt[8], by permission)

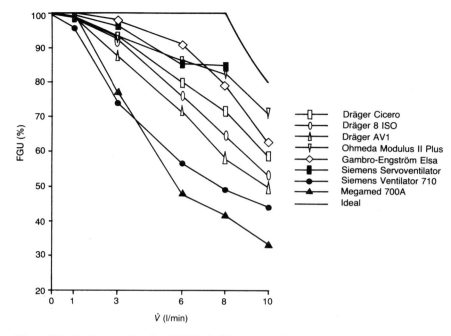

Figure 7.7 Fresh gas utilization (FGU) of different breathing systems as a function of fresh gas flow ($\dot{V}$) (From Zbinden and Feigenwinter[36], by permission)

and active control of the opening of the excess gas discharge valve[15]. In all circle absorber systems tested, a sufficiently high degree of fresh gas utilization could be gained if the fresh gas flow was decreased to 1.5 l/min or lower[36].

Equilibration will take longer, the lower the fresh gas utilization, which in turn may have an adverse effect on the course of low flow and minimal flow anaesthesia when time constants are long in any case. However, the design of the system has no influence on anaesthesia management with closed breathing systems, since there is no discharge of excess gas and fresh gas utilization amounts to 100%.

Furthermore, it must be considered that in the case of low fresh gas flow, the oxygen content of the fresh gas has to be increased in order to ensure an adequate oxygen concentration.

7.2.4.3 Specified range of operation

According to its instructions for use[15], the conventional circle absorption system 8 ISO (Drägerwerk, Lübeck, Germany) can be used both semi-closed and closed. This also applies to the compact breathing systems of the new generation of anaesthetic machines. Anaesthesia management with a closed, or virtually closed, system is specifically included in the range of operation quoted for the following anaesthetic machines: Cicero (Drägerwerk, Lübeck, Germany), Elisa, EAS 9010 and 9020 (Gambro Engström, Bromma, Sweden), Megamed 700 and Mivolan (Megamed, Cham, Switzerland)[15,20,30]. The only exception is the AV 1 anaesthetic machine (Drägerwerk, Lübeck, Germany), although it has convincingly proven its adherence to all requirements for safe performance of minimal flow anaesthesia. Without any definite restriction, the apparatus is approved 'for operation with semi-closed absorption circle system'. But a fresh gas flow of at least 1 l/min is quoted for controlled ventilation with this apparatus. This restriction of the range of operation is actually unjustified since, as long as the breathing bag (which assumes the function of a gas reservoir) is filled, ventilation is not affected in any way by the fresh gas flow.

7.2.5   Carbon dioxide absorbers

Today's common use of double carbon dioxide absorbers, containing about 1 kg absorbant each[37], or of one twin-chambered Jumbo canister, containing 2 kg absorbent, satisfies the requirements placed on all low flow techniques. Adequate absorption capacity is ensured if pelleted soda lime is used which is evaluated as being the most effective[38,39]. According to Dräger and ICI, the absorption capacity of 1 litre of soda lime amounts to at least 120 litres of carbon dioxide[40]. If the entire exhaled gas in closed system anaesthesia passes the absorber, a utilization period of about 5 h can be calculated for 1 litre of soda lime assuming a minute volume of 10 l/min and an expired carbon dioxide concentration of 4% by volume. This value also could be confirmed in laboratory tests.

7.2.5.1   Utilization period

Accordingly, a utilization period of about 5 h for the soda lime filling of a 1 litre absorber canister is unanimously quoted, at least in German textbooks. This is the reason why double absorbers are frequently used. Usually, the contents of the absorber proximal to the expiratory valve are disposed of after each working day and a newly filled absorber is fitted into the system.

The utilization periods achieved in clinical use, however, are considerably longer[41]. In accordance with the results of the author's own investigations, the utilization period of 1 litre absorber canisters ranges between 40 and 60 h if anaesthesia is performed exclusively with a comparatively high fresh gas flow of 4.4 l/min. If however, whenever possible, the flow is reduced to 0.5 l/min, the maximum time at this flow will be some 70–80% of the total use of the absorber (see Section 6.2.2). Under these conditions the utilization period of the 1 litre absorber canister decreases to around 10–15 h. The difference between the figures given in the textbooks and the measured values can be explained by the fact that, as a function of fresh gas flow and utilization, if a rebreathing system is used semi-closed only a certain part of the exhaled air really passes the absorber (see Figure 4.1). Furthermore, under clinical conditions the soda lime is not exposed continuously to the expired gas, but only intermittently. During the load-free interim periods, the absorbed carbon dioxide penetrates from the surface into the core of the soda lime granules, at which the external layers are regenerated to hydroxide. In this way the surface of the granules become available again for carbon dioxide absorption[40]. Another factor which has a specific favourable effect on the absorption capacity in performance of low flow anaesthesia is the maintenance or even increase of humidity in soda lime.

7.2.5.2 Implications for anaesthetic practice

In clinical practice, the utilization period measured for absorbers filled with pelleted soda lime is, depending on the fresh gas flow, considerably longer than that quoted in the literature. Routine disposal of the absorber filling, for instance after each working day, should be rejected particularly for reasons of ecology and economy. If the inspired and expired carbon dioxide concentration is measured continuously, anaesthesia can even be performed with a single 1 litre absorber canister, whereby the absorption capacity can be utilized completely without impairing patient safety. However, if carbon dioxide monitoring is not available, the use of double or Jumbo absorbers should be mandatory. The contents of the absorber proximal to the expiratory valve should only be discarded if the indicator of the second absorber signals the beginning of exhaustion of the soda lime[40]. The colour change of the indicator, however, cannot be taken as a very reliable sign of soda lime exhaustion, since it may be deactivated by intense ultraviolet light[42]. It is proven clinical practice to note down the filling date of the absorber on an adhesive label fixed to the canister as an additional safeguard. Even in very long-lasting anaesthetics with the flow reduced to its utmost extent, one can assume that the absorptive capacity of a newly filled double or Jumbo absorber system will be sufficient for at least the whole working day.

7.2.6 Anaesthesia ventilators

Controlled ventilation during anaesthesia with low fresh gas flow presents a number of problems which will be dealt with in detail.

7.2.6.1 Anaesthetic machines without gas reservoir

The majority of conventional anaesthesia ventilators equipped with hanging bellows fill during expiration to provide the gas volume that is delivered to the patient with the following ventilation stroke (Figure 7.8a,b). The bellows is located in a pressure chamber. Positive pressure in the bellows chamber results in compression of the bellows, so that the gas which filled the bellows during the expiratory phase is squeezed into the breathing system. During the patient's expiration the bellows is filled again with a mixture of fresh and exhaled gas. With hanging bellows, the expiratory filling of the bellows may be assisted by a weight at the bottom of the bellows (Ventilog, Drägerwerk, Lübeck). In previous types of German anaesthesia ventilators with rising bellows, expiratory filling was assisted by a negative pressure in the bellows chamber (Pulmomat, Drägerwerk, Lübeck). The filling process is completed once the bellows has reached the adjustment plate at its preselected position. Exhaled gas and fresh gas which continues to flow into the system after the bellows has reached its stop are discharged via the excess gas valve[43]. The AV-E ventilator of the Narkomed Anesthesia Systems (North American Dräger, Telford, USA) is equipped with a rising bellows, which fills due to the force of the inflowing exhaled gas (Figure 7.9). But as the expiratory

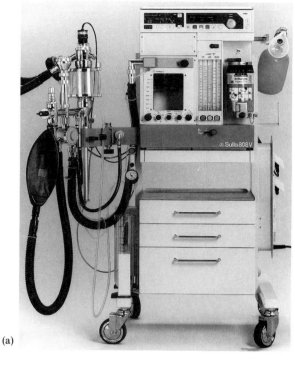

(a)

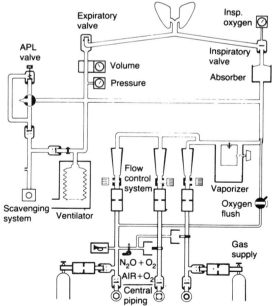

(b)

Figure 7.8   (a) Sulla 808 V anaesthetic machine (Drägerwerk, Lübeck, Germany). (b) Flow diagram of the conventional type anaesthetic machine (Sulla 808 V)

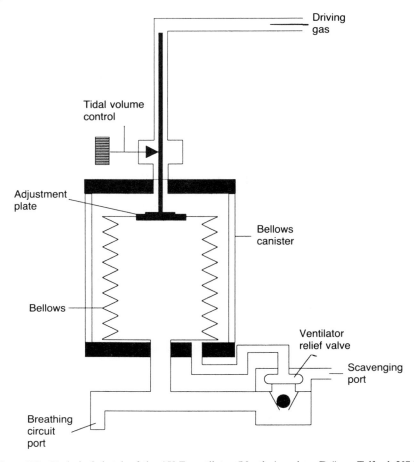

Figure 7.9   Technical sketch of the AV-E ventilator (North American Dräger, Telford, USA): the expiratory movement of the bellows is limited by the position of the adjustment plate (From Cicman et al.[12], by permission)

movement of this bellows is also limited by the position of the adjustment plate, preselected according to the desired tidal volume. In each expiratory pause the excess gas is vented into the scavenging system[12].

7.2.6.1.1   AIRWAY PRESSURE AND VENTILATION CHARACTERISTICS WITH FRESH GAS FLOW REDUCTION

If the fresh gas flow is low in such machines with forced expired filling of the bellows, there is only a comparatively small fresh gas volume available to be added to the exhaled gas filling the bellows during expiration. The breathing system is subject to negative pressure until the bellows reaches the stop. This initial negative expiratory pressure may therefore be accentuated by flow reduction, especially if the exhaled gas flows slowly back into the breathing system, for instance in patients suffering from chronic obstructive pulmonary disease[44]. However, if during the inspiratory phase the gas loss resulting from leaks and uptake is greater than the fresh gas volume fed into the system during expiration, the recirculating volume of exhaled gas will be insufficient to fill the bellows completely. In ventilators with obligatory expansion of the bellows, a transition from intermittent positive pressure ventilation (JPPV) to alternating pressure ventilation (APV) with simultaneous reduction of airway pressure and tidal volume (Figure 7.10) will be observed. The tendency of ventilation characteristics to change with flow reduction decreases as a function of the gas tightness of anaesthesia ventilators and takes place in the following order: Pulmomat, Spiromat, Ventilog (Drägerwerk, Lübeck, Germany). A desired positive end-expiratory pressure (PEEP) can only be achieved in these machines under conditions of flow reduction, if a sufficient amount of excess gas volume is maintained in an adequately leakproof system (Figures 7.11a,c). In the AV-E ventilator (North American Dräger, Telford, USA), fresh gas deficiency will result in an insufficient expiratory filling of the bellows, a decrease of the peak pressure and the tidal volume, but will not change the ventilatory pattern. All these different ventilators have in common that there is no additional reserve of gas volume. Whenever there is any gas volume deficiency resulting from an imbalance between gas loss via uptake and leakages and the fresh gas volume, an immediate alteration of the ventilation parameters will occur.

According to Spieß[46], the increased demands with respect to leakproofness of conventional-type anaesthesia ventilators can be met by control of the PEEP valve. To proceed in this manner means that, during performance of low flow anaesthesia, the unwanted expiratory discharge of anaesthetic gas via the excess gas discharge valve, opening at 2 mbar, can be reduced. This will be possible in those ventilators in which the PEEP valve is switched into the excess gas outlet. A PEEP can be only achieved in these machines if an adequate gas volume is available. In this case it may be necessary to readjust the PEEP valve control, an adjustment actually intended only to enhance the leakproofness of the ventilator.

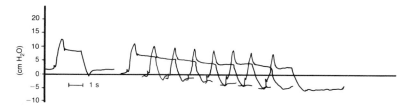

Figure 7.10   Course of the pressure within the breathing system at a fresh gas flow of 0.5 l/min and an actual leakage of 150 ml/min. Decrease of inspired peak and plateau pressure and transition to alternating pressure ventilation. Fresh gas deficiency results in considerable alteration of the ventilation pattern if the expiratory expansion of the bellows is assisted by an additional force (From Baum and Schneider[45])

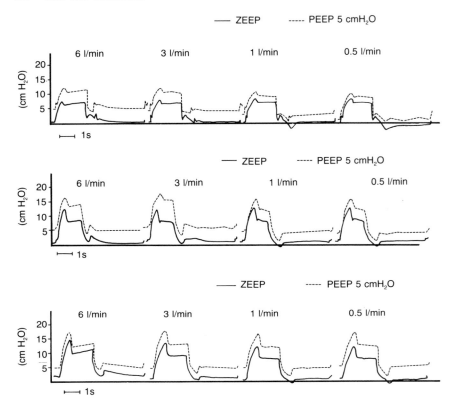

Figure 7.11 Pressure within the breathing system during one ventilatory cycle, as a function of different fresh gas flows ($\dot{V}$). (a) Pulmomat 19.1: with decreasing $\dot{V}$, transition to alternating pressure ventilation, a preset PEEP cannot be attained. (b) Spiromat 650: with decreasing $\dot{V}$, decrease of inspired peak and plateau pressure, a preset PEEP cannot be built up to the extent selected. (c) Ventilog: with decreasing $\dot{V}$, only negligible decrease of inspired peak and plateau pressure, the preset PEEP will attain the desired level. ZEEP: zero end expiratory pressure (From
Baum and Schneider[45])

7.2.6.1.2   BREATHING VOLUMES WITH FRESH GAS FLOW REDUCTION

Where conventional anaesthetic machines with continuous flow are concerned, the breathing volume is a function of the fresh gas flow. In addition to the volume supplied by the inspiratory compression of the bellows, the fresh gas volume flowing into the breathing system during inspiration is also applied to the patient with each inspiratory stroke. This may be explained by taking the Ventilog anaesthetic ventilator (Drägerwerk, Lübeck, Germany) as an example. The calibration of the device is designed for a fresh gas flow of 4 l/min. Given a minute volume of 7000 ml, a respiratory frequency of 10 per minute, and an inspiratory–expiratory ratio I:E = 1:2, the machine-supplied stroke volume of 567 ml and an inspired fresh gas volume of 133 ml add up to the tidal volume of 700 ml. If the fresh gas flow is reduced to

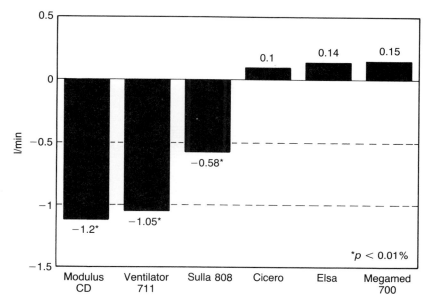

Figure 7.12   Change in minute volume (MV) with reduction of fresh gas flow: average values of differences in minute volumes, measured immediately prior to, and 15 min after reduction of fresh gas flow from 4.4 to 0.5 l/min. Whenever the fresh gas is fed into the breathing system continuously, the MV will decrease significantly with flow reduction

0.5 l/min, the volume fed into the system during inspiration is reduced to 17 ml, so that, together with the machine-supplied stroke volume, the breathing volume amounts to only 584 ml. Mathematically, the minute volume thus decreases by 1160 ml if the flow is reduced from 4.0 to 0.5 l/min (Figure 7.12). This phenomenon is referred to in the supplement to the instructions for use of the Sulla 808 under the heading 'Possibility of metering low fresh gas volumes', as well as in other publications[15,47–49].

The interdependence between minute volume and fresh gas flow can be corrected by increasing the tidal volume set at the machine according to and at the same time as flow reduction.

7.2.6.2   Anaesthetic machines with gas reservoir

7.2.6.2.1   VENTILATORS WITH FLOATING BELLOWS

Machines of the Air-Shields Ventilator type (Figure 7.13) with rising bellows are the technical alternative to ventilators equipped with suspended bellows. The bellows of this machine are installed standing upright in the pressure chamber. It features an extremely high compliance and its expiratory filling is effected exclusively by the inflow of the fresh gas and the exhaled gas volume. During inspiration, the driving gas flows into the bellows canister in accordance with the ventilation parameters selected, and squeezes the bellows. Generally, the bellows are not completely compressed, but oscillate at an average filling level during the ventilation cycles. Imbalances between

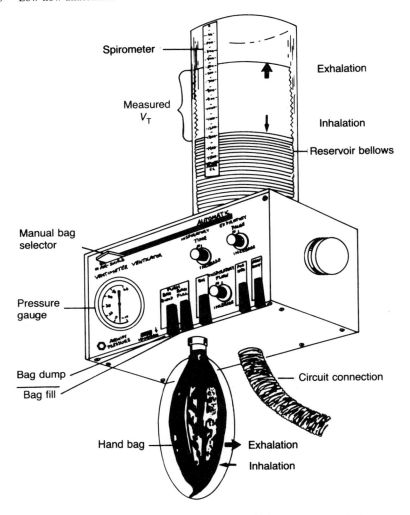

Figure 7.13   Air-Shields Ventilator with rising bellows, which serve as anaesthetic gas reservoir. (From Lowe and Ernst[50], by permission)

the fresh gas volume and the volume loss via uptake and leakages are compensated by a greater or lesser inspiratory emptying of the bellows. Thus, the floating bellows serve as an anaesthetic gas reservoir to cover the required gas supply over a certain period of time during which adequate corrections at the flow control system can be made[50]. The tidal volume can be read from the amplitude of the bellows movement. Nevertheless, the continuous flow of fresh gas into the breathing system results in the interdependence between tidal and fresh gas volume mentioned above[47]. The Ohmeda 7800 Ventilator (Ohmeda, Hatfield, UK), for instance, conforms to this type of ventilator with standing bellows. Without adequate adjustment of the

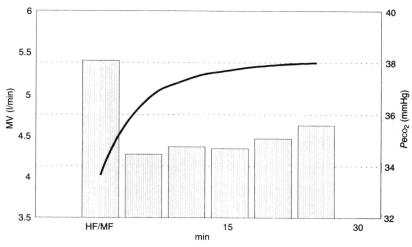

Figure 7.14   Increase of the expiratory carbon dioxide partial pressure (curve) due to decrease of minute volume (bars) resulting from fresh gas flow reduction. HF/MF: reduction of the flow from 4.4 to 0.5 l/min (Modulus CD, Ohmeda, Hatfield, UK)

ventilator settings, the fresh gas flow reduction will result in considerable alteration of the minute volume with corresponding change in the expired carbon dioxide concentration (Figure 7.14). In the manual of the Ohmeda Modulus CD, a formula is given to calculate the fresh gas volume V_{if} which is fed into the breathing system during inspiration:

$$V_{if} = \dot{V}_f/(r \times (1 + \text{E:I}))$$

where $\dot{V}_f$ = total fresh gas flow (l/min)
$\quad r$ = ventilation rate (min^{-1})
$\quad$ E:I = expiratory–inspiratory ratio

7.2.6.2.2   ANAESTHETIC MACHINES WITH GAS RESERVOIR AND DISCONTINUOUS FRESH GAS SUPPLY

With the alternative technical concepts of some anaesthetic machines such as AV 1, Cato, Cicero, Sulla 909 (Drägerwerk, Lübeck, Germany), Dogma (Heyer, Bad Ems, Germany)[51], Megamed 700 and Mirolan (Megamed, Cham, Switzerland), the tidal volume no longer depends on the fresh gas flow. All these devices are anaesthetic ventilators, which provide the gas volume for the following ventilation stroke during expiration. The AV 1, Dogma and Megamed 700 operate with conventional hanging bellows, while in the Cato and Cicero machines the ventilator is a piston pump with rolling seal. During inspiration, the fresh gas is stored in an anaesthetic gas reservoir – the manual bag – and is discontinuously fed into the system, during the expiratory phase only (Figure 7.15a,b). During expiration, the ventilator's volume is filled up from this gas reservoir and the exhaled gas that flows back into the system. As long as the reservoir itself is appropriately filled, the tidal volume (see Figure 7.12), and the ventilation pattern (Figure 7.16) remain unaffected by

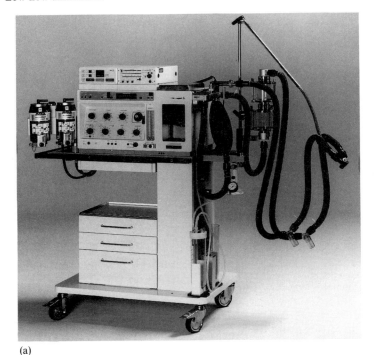

(a)

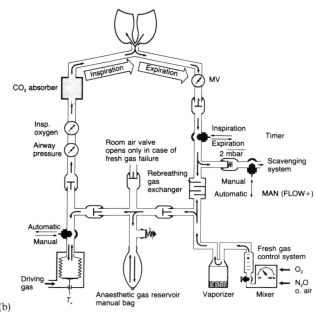

(b)

Figure 7.15   (a) AV 1 anaesthetic machine (Drägerwerk, Lübeck, Germany). (b) Flow diagram of the AV 1. Technical feature: discontinuous flow of fresh gas into the system. During inspiration, the fresh gas is stored in the manual bag, which serves as an anaesthetic gas reservoir, and is fed into the system only during expiration

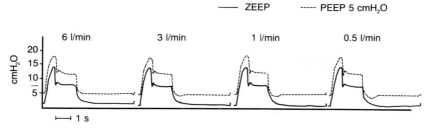

Figure 7.16   Pressure within the circle system during one ventilatory cycle, as a function of different fresh gas flows. The airway pressure remains completely unchanged, and the desired PEEP is attained independent of the fresh gas flow (From Baum and Schneider[45])

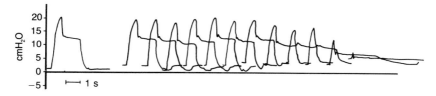

Figure 7.17   The AV 1 anaesthetic machine. Course of the pressure within the breathing system with a fresh gas flow of 0.5 l/min and an actual leakage of 150 ml/min: decrease of the inspired peak and plateau pressure with simultaneous increase of expiratory pressure (From Baum and Schneider[45])

the setting of the fresh gas flow. A preset PEEP is built up reliably and maintained even with the lowest possible fresh gas flows. If the breathing bag is emptied completely and collapses totally in the expiratory phase, the ventilator will no longer be adequately filled and both minute volume and airway pressure decrease. Such a malfunction will be signalled instantly, if the alarm limits for airway pressure and minute volume are adjusted appropriately. Where the Cato and Cicero (Drägerwerk, Lübeck, Germany) are concerned, a clear text alarm message 'fresh gas deficiency' signals this problem immediately.

7.2.6.2.3   MACHINE-SPECIFIC FEATURES

The following particular features were observed in clinical use of the machines:

AV 1 (Drägerwerk, Lübeck, Germany) (Figure 7.15a,b). With a leakage loss of 150 l/min, simulated by continuously extracting this gas volume from the system, positive pressure builds up in the system in spite of the resulting gas deficiency (Figure 7.17). Since the expiratory expansion of the ventilator bellows is assisted by a weight, one would expect a negative pressure in the system in case of volume deficiency, as the bellows cannot reach the stop. However, due to the specific design, the negative pressure resulting from bellows expansion acts as a closing force upon the expiratory valve. The

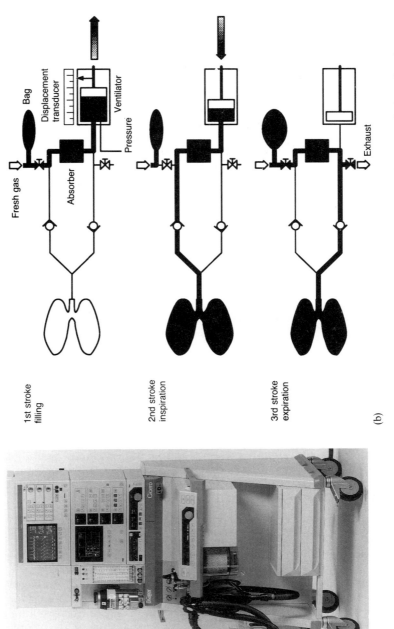

Figure 7.18 (a) Cicero anaesthetic workstation (Drägerwerk, Lübeck, Germany). (b) Flow diagram of the Cicero anaesthetic workstation

patient hose system is thus closed against the breathing system, which in turn causes the build-up of a PEEP in the patient system. Nevertheless, the inadequate filling of the bellows results in a decrease in tidal volume, accompanied by a corresponding drop in peak ventilation pressure. After a certain delay, the machine will switch to alternating pressure ventilation as expected.

Cicero (Drägerwerk, Lübeck, Germany) (Figure 7.18a,b). The Cicero anaesthesia workstation features high-grade leakproofness which is checked by automatically performed sequences of self-tests when the unit is switched on. The ventilator permits ventilation even with extremely low tidal volumes down to 20 ml. Fresh gas utilization is optimized by exact timing and control of the valve function during each expiratory phase. When the ventilator piston starts to move back, the valve to the fresh gas reservoir is opened prior to the expiratory valve. This means that the gas, filling the ventilator, contains the greatest possible proportion of fresh gas, whereas when the excess gas discharge valve is opened it is primarily exhaled gas which is released as waste. The leakproofness of the system is enhanced in so far as the excess gas discharge valve is not opened passively, as is the case with conventional systems, but opening of this valve at an end-expiratory pressure of more than $0.1\,\text{kPa}$ ($\simeq 1\,\text{cmH}_2\text{O}$) is due to active control of the valve. The excess gas discharge valve is closed again if the pressure drops below $0.05\,\text{kPa}$ ($\simeq 0.5\,\text{cmH}_2\text{O}$). This ensures that excess gas can only be discharged if the breathing system is filled sufficiently. In this way the opening of the system is automatically adapted to the fresh gas flow. Fresh gas deficiency does not result in negative pressure within the breathing system, since the

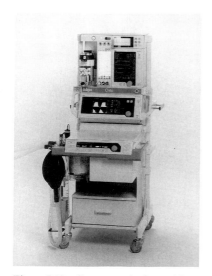

Figure 7.19 Cato anaesthetic machine (Drägerwerk, Lübeck, Germany)

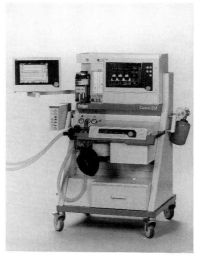

Figure 7.20 Cicero EM anaesthetic workstation (Drägerwerk, Lübeck, Germany)

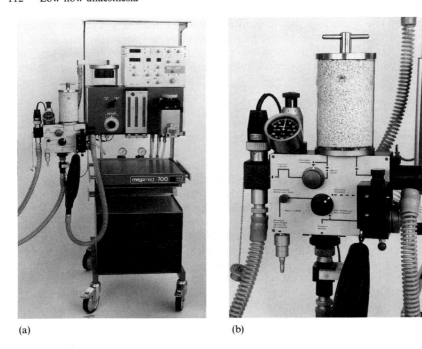

(a)   (b)

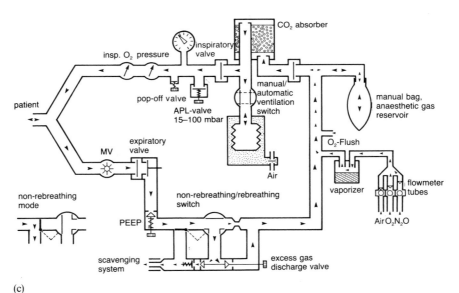

(c)

Figure 7.21   (a) Megamed 700 anaesthetic machine (Megamed, Cham, Switzerland). (b) Compact circle absorber system of the Megamed 700. Technical feature: the excess gas discharge valve has to be set manually; a switch enables a change from rebreathing to non-rebreathing mode. (c) Flow diagram of the Megamed 700: the manual bag serves as an anaesthetic gas reservoir; discontinuous fresh gas supply into the system during expiratory phase only

return of the ventilator piston is interrupted immediately, and the problem is signalled at the machine's front panel display by clear text message. The same features characterizing this ventilator and the breathing system apply to the Cato (Figure 7.19) and the Cicero EM (Figure 7.20) anaesthetic machines (Drägerwerk, Lübeck, Germany). With the Cicero EM, a high grade of integration of monitoring and controls will be gained. All settings are performed by a rotating knob.

Megamed 700 (Megamed, Cham, Switzerland) (Figure 7.21a–c). In the Megamed 700 anaesthetic machine the excess gas is not discharged from the system during the expiratory phase via an automatically opening valve. The opening of the excess gas discharge valve must be adapted manually to the selected fresh gas flow and has to be adjusted so as to ensure a sufficient filling of the reservoir bag. The reservoir bag collapses once the valve is opened too wide, the bellows of the ventilator is no longer adequately filled and the tidal volume decreases. If, however, the valve is closed too much, the reservoir bag is completely filled and a positive pressure builds up in the breathing system. Particular attention must be paid to correct manual adjustment of this valve if the fresh gas flow is changed. Correct adjustment of the APL valve to a value 10 mbar above peak pressure[30] prevents accidental barotrauma. The Megamed breathing system type 048NR can be switched from rebreathing to non-rebreathing mode. The entire volume of exhaled gas is discharged from the system in this mode, and the fresh gas volume must at the least correspond to the minute volume. If this mode is selected, concentration changes in the breathing system proceed rapidly, accelerating wash-in and wash-out processes considerably. The tidal volume can be set independently of the fresh gas flow, as the fresh gas is fed into the system only during the expiratory phase, whereas during inspiration the fresh gas is stored in the manual bag serving as the anaesthetic gas reservoir. The newest anaesthetic machine from the Megamed company, Mivolan, can be optionally equipped with an excess gas discharge valve which opens automatically.

Modulus CD (Ohmeda, Hatfield, UK) (Figure 7.22a,b). The Modulus CD anaesthetic workstation is suitable for the performance of anaesthesia even with lowest fresh gas flows. The flow control unit allows precise and easy adjustment even in the low flow range. Oxygen and nitrous oxide controls are connected by a chain, thus making it impossible to adjust a fresh gas oxygen concentration lower than 25% (Figure 7.22b). The Link 25 anti-hypoxic device does not hinder the precise setting of very low gas flows. The compact mini-absorber system (MAS) proved to be highly gas tight. Comprehensive monitoring devices facilitate safe performance of anaesthesia. Computerized automatic record keeping is possible, as all data can be stored at short intervals on a diskette with the aid of the built-in disk drive. The floating rising bellows of the ventilator serve as an anaesthetic gas reservoir, by which small imbalances between the fresh gas volume and the gas loss via leakages and uptake can be compensated. As the fresh gas is fed into the breathing system continuously, the tidal volume being supplied to the patient is dependent upon the fresh gas flow. The technical concept of the Excel anaesthetic machine is identical to that of the Modulus CD.

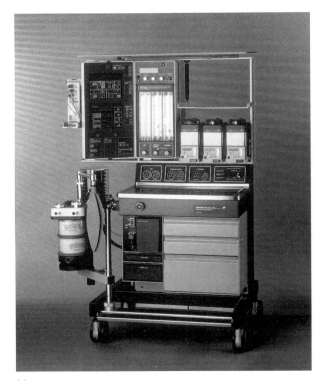

(a)

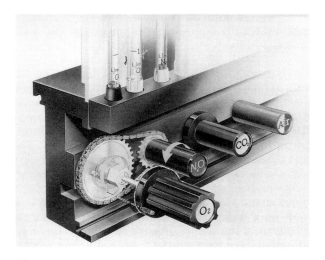

(b)

Figure 7.22   (a) Modulus CD anaesthetic workstation (Ohmeda, Hatfield, UK). (b) Anti-hypoxic safety device Link 25: oxygen and nitrous oxide controls are linked by a chain

Narkomed 4 (North American Dräger, Telford, USA). The Narkomed 4 workstation also offers comprehensive monitoring for safe performance of anaesthesia and computerized automatic record-keeping. However, the technical features of the flow control system, the breathing system and the anaesthesia ventilator are more conventional. The fresh gas flow is fed into the breathing system continuously, resulting in a dependency of fresh gas flow and inspired volume in the case of controlled ventilation. There is no anaesthetic gas reservoir available, as the expiratory expansion of the rising bellows is stopped by the preset position of the adjustment plate. Only if this stop is adjusted to its highest position at the top of the bellows canister can the ventilator be used with floating bellows which then may serve as a anaesthetic gas reservoir. Though the breathing system featured a high number of connections, it proved to be adequately gas tight. However, the anti-hypoxic safety device of the flow control system, the oxygen ratio controller (ORC), is so sensitive, that precise control of the oxygen and nitrous oxide flow even in the range of low flow anaesthesia is nearly impossible and needs frequent corrections.

SA 2 (Drägerwerk, Lübeck, Germany) (Figure 7.23a,b). The SA 2 belongs to that type of anaesthetic machine in which the fresh gas is fed into the system only during the expiratory phase. During inspiration, the gas is stored in the manual bag, which thus functions as an anaesthetic gas reservoir. If equipped with two flowmeter tubes each for oxygen and nitrous oxide, the flow control system allows precise adjustment of gas flows down to $0.1\,l/min$. The pneumatically controlled ORC, however, impedes adjustment of the oxygen flow to values lower than $0.35\,l/min$. The compact breathing system, CU 1, is highly gas tight with a mean leakage loss lower than $50\,ml/min$ at $4\,kPa$ ($\simeq 40\,cmH_2O$). The APL valve has to be adapted carefully to the airway pressure, otherwise an inspiratory gas loss may occur. In the event of gas deficiency and resultant negative pressure within the system during expiratory expansion of the bellows, room air is entrained into the system via the auxiliary valve which opens at -200 to $-400\,Pa$ ($\simeq 2$–$4\,cmH_2O$). In the CU 1 breathing system, the absorber is directly attached to the system being connected into the expiratory limb. Optionally the machine is available with the absorber in the inspiratory limb in order to avoid water condensation within the CU 1 breathing system, which may be advantageous in low flow anaesthesia. The RA 2 ventilator is electrically driven and equipped with a hanging bellows. The poor performance of the ORC in the low flow range is the deciding factor for the limited suitability of the SA 2 machine in using very low fresh gas flows. The anaesthetic machine SA 2, however, meets all the requirements for safe and simple performance of low flow anaesthesia.

Servo Anaesthesia System (Siemens-Elema, Solna, Sweden) (Figure 7.24a,b). The Servo Ventilator C and D equipped with an Anaesthesia Circle System 985 belongs to the group of machines featuring gas reservoir and discontinuous fresh gas supply into the system. The fresh gas is mixed by a blender and, having passed the Siemens vaporizer (of the jet vaporizer type[21]), it is fed into the system at defined volumes only during inspiration. Following carbon dioxide absorption, the recirculating exhaled air is mixed with the fresh gas during the inspiratory stroke of the ventilator. The ventilator with

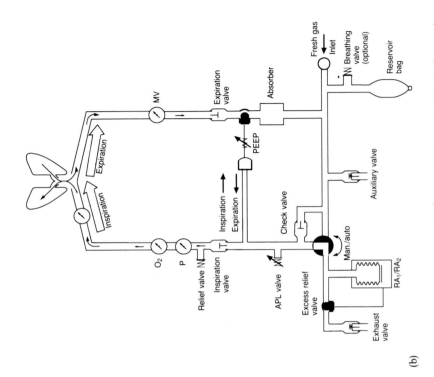

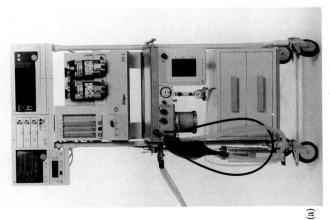

Figure 7.23 (a) SA 2 anaesthetic machine with **RA 1/RA 2** electric ventilator and CU 1 breathing system (Drägerwerk, Lübeck, Germany). (b) Flow diagram of the SA 2 anaesthetic machine

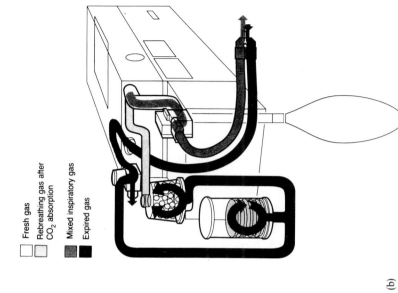

Fresh gas

Rebreathing gas after CO_2 absorption

Mixed inspiratory gas

Expired gas

(b)

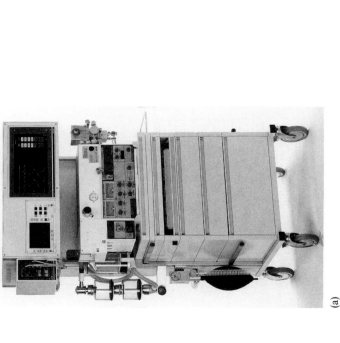

(a)

Figure 7.24 (a) Siemens Servo Ventilator with Anaesthetic Circle System 985 (Siemens-Elema, Solna, Sweden). (b) Flow diagram of the Siemens Servo Ventilator with Anaesthetic Circle System 985. Technical feature: discontinuous inspired supply of fresh gas, anaesthetic ventilator with rising bellows

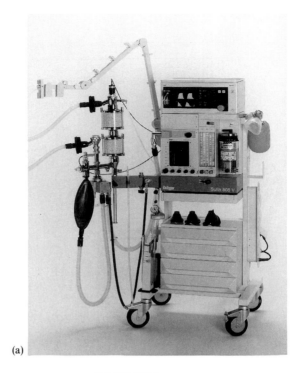

(a)

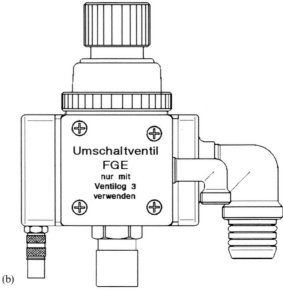

Umschaltventil
FGE
nur mit
Ventilog 3
verwenden

(b)

Figure 7.25 (a) Sulla 808 anaesthetic machine equipped with FGE valve and Ventilog 3 (Drägerwerk, Lübeck, Germany). (b) Fresh gas decoupling valve (FGE valve). (c) Flow diagram of the Sulla 808 with FGE valve. Technical feature: during inspiration the fresh gas flows into the manual bag, which serves as an anaesthetic gas reservoir

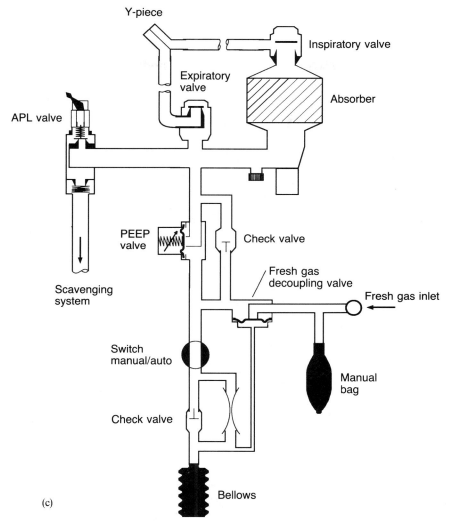

(c)

rising bellows corresponds to the type of the Air Shields Ventilator, the floating bellows serving as a as reservoir. According to the author's own experience, the flow transducer measuring the expired gas volume was extremely susceptible to malfunction, which was attributable to the frequently observed contamination of the sensor. Such contamination occurred in particular when leakage losses had to be compensated for by frequent actuation of the 'gas exchange button'. The leak test of this machine was cumbersome, as it could not be performed under resting conditions but only if the ventilator was working. For adequate performance, the machine needed at least a fresh gas flow of 0.7 to 0.8 l/min.

Sulla 808 equipped with fresh gas decoupling (FGE) valve and the anaesthetic ventilator Ventilog 3 (Drägerwerk, Lübeck, Germany) (Figure 7.25a–c). The

FGE valve is an additional device which can be attached to the circle absorber system 8 or 9 ISO. It is connected to the conventional ventilator, Ventilog 3, by two tubes needed for pneumatic control of the fresh gas flow and the PEEP valve. During inspiration, the fresh gas is temporarily stored in the manual bag which serves as a gas reservoir, and is fed into the breathing system only during the expiratory phase. The anaesthetist, however, has to observe carefully the performance of the valve. Following thermo-disinfection with a washing machine, water may accumulate within the FGE valve or the control tubes, resulting in dangerous malfunction of this device. Alternating PEEP levels or even severe obstruction of the expiratory flow were observed. It cannot be overemphasized that this device should preferably be autoclaved and dried carefully after daily use. Provided that this procedure and carefully performed leak test are carried out, the Sulla 800 and 808 anaesthesia machines with FGE valve meet the technical requirements for low and even minimal flow anaesthesia.

7.2.6.2.4   BAG-IN-BOTTLE VENTILATORS

Elsa, EAS 9010 and EAS 9020 (Gambro-Engström, Bromma, Sweden) (Figure 7.26a,b). The Elsa anaesthetic machine operates with a classic bag-in-bottle ventilator. The 4-litre patient bag, which is placed in a pressure chamber, is filled with fresh gas and exhaled air during expiration. During inspiration, driving gas flows into the pressure chamber in accordance with the set ventilation parameters, the bag is squeezed and part of its gas volume is delivered into the breathing system. In spite of the fact that the fresh gas is fed into the system continuously, the ventilation is not influenced by the rate of the fresh gas flow. The inspired flow is measured electronically and the inspiration phase is completed once the set tidal volume has been supplied to the patient. The time cycle of the ventilator's control thus changes as a function of the fresh gas flow selected. Possible imbalances between fresh gas volume and gas loss via uptake and leaks are compensated by greater or lesser evacuation of the patient bag. The tidal volume only decreases if this gas reservoir is no longer filled sufficiently. In the event of fresh gas deficiency, the unit signals the message 'patient bag empty' on the alarm display. The compact breathing system is highly gas tight, and a leak test is performed automatically. The electronic vaporizer can be set to a maximum output of 8%. To facilitate precise adjustment of the gas flows in the low flow range, the electronic flowmeter bar graph display can be switched to high resolution. Thus, the Elsa anaesthetic machine meets all requirements for performance of anaesthesia with even the lowest fresh gas flows. The newer Gambro-Engström anaesthetic machines EAS 9010 and 9020 (Figure 7.27) are equipped with comprehensive monitoring in accordance with the requirements of the draft of the common European standard prEN 740. Special technical features of the EAS 9020 are a battery back-up power supply and a direct connection between the manual bag and the breathing system (Figure 7.28), whereas in the other machines squeezing of this bag acts indirectly by an increase of the pressure in the pressure chamber.

Anesthesia System 711 (Siemens-Elema, Solna, Sweden) (Figure 7.29a,b). Contrary to the Servo Anaesthesia System mentioned beforehand, the Anesthesia System 711 is a more conventional type of machine. It is equipped

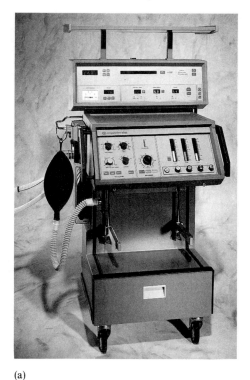

(a)

(b)

Figure 7.26 (a) Elsa anaesthetic machine (Gambro-Engström, Bromma, Sweden). (b) Flow diagram of the Elsa. Technical features: electronic metering system for volatile anaesthetics, bag-in-bottle ventilator

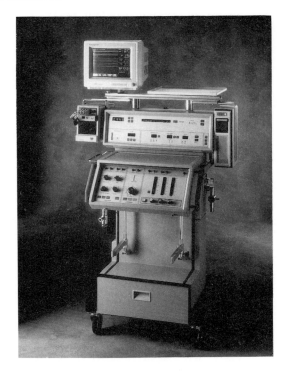

Figure 7.27   EAS 9010 anaesthetic workstation (Gambro-Engström, Bromma, Sweden)

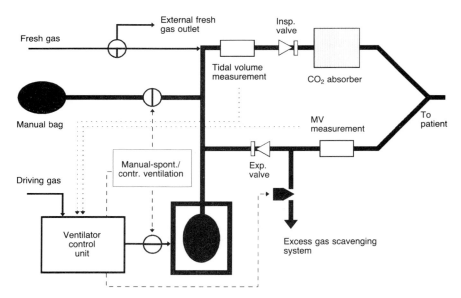

Figure 7.28   Flow diagram of the anaesthetic workstation EAS 9020 (Gambro-Engström, Bromma, Sweden). Technical feature: the manual bag is connected directly to the breathing system

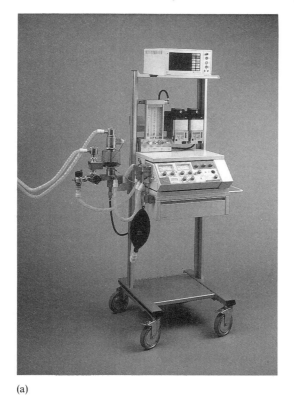

(a)

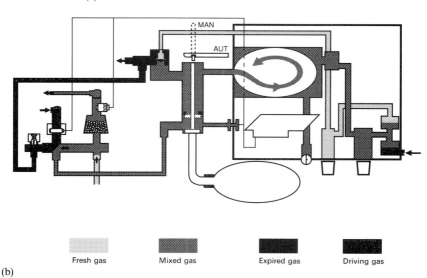

| Fresh gas | Mixed gas | Expired gas | Driving gas |

(b)

Figure 7.29   (a) Siemens Anesthesia System 711 (Siemens-Elema, Solna, Sweden). (b) Flow diagram of the Siemens Anesthesia System 711. Technical feature: a conventional machine with a bag-in-bottle ventilator

Table 7.1   Volumes (in litres) of some newer anaesthetic machines

	AV 1	Cicero	Elsa	Megamed	Sulla
Patient hose system	0.9	0.9	0.9	0.9	0.9
Breathing system	1.2	0.6	0.4	0.5	0.4
Absorber	1.0	2.0	1.0	1.0	1.0
Anaesthetic gas reservoir	1.5	1.5	3.0	1.5	–
Hose connections	0.8	0.5	0.4	0.4	0.5
Ventilator volume	0.7	0.7	–	0.7	0.7
Total volume	6.1	6.2	5.7	5.0	3.5

with a commonly used flow control system and plenum vaporizers, and the fresh gas is fed into the system continuously. The anaesthetic ventilator is a classic bag-in-bottle design, with a 3-litre patient bag. Thus, a sufficient amount of reservoir gas is available for initial compensation of gas volume imbalances. With this device, flow reduction down to 0.5 l/min could be realized in clinical practice.

7.2.7   System volumes

With constant uptake and fresh gas flow, the time constant is directly proportional to the volume of the entire gas-filled space (see Section 5.2.3). It is calculated from the sum of machine-related gas volumes and functional residual capacity. With high system volumes the time constant is long, and correspondingly short with small system volumes.

Table 7.1 lists the volumes of some newer anaesthesia machines. This compilation is based on the following conditions: the patient system consists of two corrugated hoses of 1 m length, only one 1 litre or one Jumbo absorber canister is fitted in the breathing system and the anaesthetic gas reservoirs – the 4-litre patient bag of the Elsa machine, and the 2.3-litre manual bag of the machines AV 1, Cicero or Megamed – are only filled up to 75% of their maximum capacity. Under these conditions, the machine-related gas volume can be assumed to be 5.3 litres on average. Together with a functional residual capacity of 2.5 litres, the volume of the entire gas-filled space adds up to 7.8 litres.

For an adult patient of 75 kg body weight, an uptake of about 0.4 l/min can be assumed 30 min after induction of anaesthesia. Given a fresh gas flow of 4.4 l/min, the time constant then amounts to about 2 min; with a flow of 0.5 l/min it is 78 min. In spite of the possibly very small dimensions of some compact breathing systems, the apparatus gas space of the new generation of anaesthetic machines is large enough that, with a flow reduction from 4.4 l/min to 0.5 l/min, the time constant increases by a factor of approximately 40.

7.3   Anaesthetic machines with closed breathing system

By definition, in closed system anaesthesia only that volume of fresh gas is fed into the system which just replenishes the losses resulting from the uptake and possible leaks. A fundamental problem with this technique is the continuous adaptation of fresh gas composition and its volume to the changing uptake during the course of anaesthesia (see Section 4.3). This method cannot be performed with anaesthetic machines without a gas reservoir, since precise adaptation to the respective uptake is virtually impossible in spite of very careful and frequent readjustment of the flow control system and the vaporizer. Furthermore, if machines without a gas reservoir are used, immediate changes in ventilation patterns occur whenever the fresh gas volume does not exactly meet the actual gas loss.

Although possible imbalances between the set fresh gas flow and gas losses can be compensated by variable filling of the gas reservoir with such anaesthetic machines, continuous manual adjustments of the fresh gas flow and its composition are not practicable in clinical routine.

An alternative to conventional gas dosage is to regulate the substitution of the gas volume loss by means of electronic feedback control[52-55]. Although the concepts for such electronic control are quite well developed and prototypes of these machines were already in clinical use[55], at present there is only one anaesthetic machine of this type commercially available.

7.3.1 The PhysioFlex anaesthetic machine

The PhysioFlex anaesthetic machine (Physio Medical Systems BV, Haarlem, The Netherlands), was developed by scientists and engineers of Rotterdam University under the chairmanship of W. Erdmann (Figure 7.30a,b). It uses an entirely new technical concept[56]. The ventilator consists of four membrane chambers connected in parallel, with a capacity of 625 ml each. Depending on the selected tidal volume, one or several chambers are simultaneously switched into the system. The breathing system itself is valveless. Driven by a blower, the anaesthetic gas circulates within the system continuously at a flow of 70 l/min. If driving gas is fed into the external part of the activated membrane chambers, the membranes are compressed, which causes ventilation of the patient. The movement of the metallic membranes is measured capacitively, whereby the ventilation volume is checked. The concentration of oxygen is continuously measured paramagnetically and that of the volatile anaesthetic, of nitrous oxide and carbon dioxide by means of infrared absorption. Oxygen and nitrous oxide are fed into the system via electronically controlled metering systems, whereby the oxygen is proportioned such that the preselected oxygen concentration is maintained constant. The volume of nitrous oxide fed into the system is adequate to keep the volume in the breathing system constant. This is verified by capacitive measurement of the expiratory filling of the membrane chambers. The chosen volatile anaesthetic is injected into the system in liquid form by a syringe driven by a stepper motor at such a rate that a desired expiratory concentration is attained rapidly and maintained constant at this level. Since the anaesthetic gas is circulating continuously within the system, the liquid anaesthetic evaporates quickly so that the gas concentration in the entire system is rapidly equalized. Rapid decrease in the anaesthetic concentration is achieved by switching a charcoal filter into the circulating gas (Figure 7.30b: VA filter). If the foreign gas concentration in the system exceeds a value of 10% by volume, a 2-minutes flushing phase with high fresh gas flow is requested at the monitor.

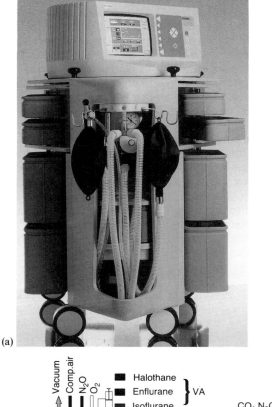

(a)

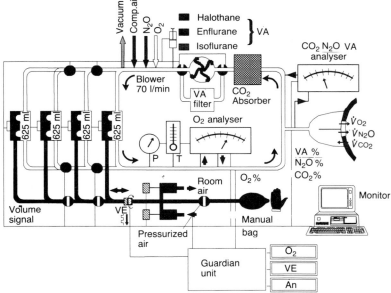

(b)

Figure 7.30   (a) PhysioFlex anaesthetic machine (Physio, Haarlem, The Netherlands). (b) Flow diagram of the PhysioFlex: anaesthetic machine with closed rebreathing system and electronic closed-loop feedback control of anaesthetic gas supply

The time constant of this system is very short due to the technical features mentioned. All data and measured values, including the gas volumes fed into the system, are displayed on a monitor screen and can be transferred for further processing to a computer by means of a communication program via a serial interface. Rolly proved, on the basis of mass spectrometric investigations in clinical use of this anaesthetic machine, that preselected anaesthetic gas compositions can reliably be attained and maintained with the aid of the electronically closed loop feedback control[24].

The performance of the electronic feedback control is supervised by a second measurement device, the 'guardian unit'. With the new software update, the anaesthetist will be able to switch to a second working mode, in which an excess volume of anaesthetic gas can be supplied to the patient while maintaining the preselected inspiratory composition. This mode will facilitate the management of all situations in which anaesthetic gas is needed in excess, such as the induction of small children with a face mask, where leakages often are unavoidable.

7.4   Implications for anaesthetic practice

7.4.1   Closed system anaesthesia

Quantitative closed system anaesthesia calls for electronically controlled gas and anaesthetic metering by means of closed loop feedback control. Until now, this dosage principle is only achieved in the PhysioFlex anaesthetic machine (Physio, Haarlem, Netherlands). Non-quantitative closed system anaesthesia can be performed with all those machines which satisfy the following requirements: the breathing systems must be sufficiently gas tight, flow control systems must permit the accurate adjustment of even the lowest gas flows, vaporizers must work reliably in the low flow range, and comprehensive monitoring of the anaesthetic gas composition must be ensured. These requirements are satisfied, for instance, by the Cicero, Cato and Cicero EM (Drägerwerk, Lübeck, Germany), EAS 9010 and 9020 (Gambro-Engström, Bromma, Sweden), Modulus CD (Ohmeda, Hatfield, UK) and Megamed 700 or Mivolan (Megamed, Cham, Switzerland).

7.4.2   Minimal flow anaesthesia

Although the fresh gas flow is reduced to the greatest possible extent in using semi-closed rebreathing systems, minimal flow anaesthesia is performed with a certain excess gas volume and adjustment of standardized fresh gas compositions. This procedure can be adopted in clinical practice without any problems if the following requirements are satisfied: starting with a gas flow of 100 ml/min, oxygen and nitrous oxide must be adjustable in increments of 50 ml, and the flow of already pre-mixed fresh gas to a rate of at least 500 ml/min. Furthermore, the vaporizers must work reliably at a flow of 500 ml/min, and the breathing systems must be adequately leakproof. The performance of this technique is considerably facilitated by discontinuous fresh gas supply and availability of a gas reservoir, since imbalances in volume can be compensated for and ventilation volume is then independent of the fresh gas flow. These requirements are satisfied by the following anaesthetic machines: Cicero, Cato, Cicero EM, EAS 9010 and 9020, Modulus CD and Megamed 700. However, the AV 1 and the Sulla 808 FGE (Drägerwerk, Lübeck, Germany), the Excel (Ohmeda, Hatfield, UK), the Elsa (Gambro-Engström, Bromma, Sweden) and the Anesthesia Ventilator 711 (Siemens-Elema, Solna, Sweden) have also convincingly proven adequate performance in the clinical application of this method. Restricting the operation range of the AV 1 ventilator to a flow of at least 1 l/min by the manufacturer is not really justified.

Besides continuous measurement of inspired oxygen concentration, airway pressure and minute volume, monitoring of the volatile agent concentration within the breathing system should be regarded as indispensable, since accidental over- or underdosage of the anaesthetic may be caused by a change from low to high fresh gas flows.

With careful maintenance, the technique can also be adopted for the conventional anaesthetic machines like the Sulla 808 V (Drägerwerk, Lübeck, Germany). However, this calls for increased vigilance and a sound understanding of the fundamental uptake mechanisms and of the technical function of the anaesthetic machine, since ventilation is linked to the fresh gas flow by the continuous inflow of fresh gas into the breathing system, and due to the lack of a gas reservoir. It is self-evident that the requirements placed on leakproofness must also be satisfied in these machines.

Minimal flow anaesthesia, the low flow technique with the greatest possible flow reduction in the use of semi-closed rebreathing systems, can reliably be performed in clinical practice with the new generation of anaesthetic machines. This is why the following chapters are primarily focused upon the practical performance of this technique only.

7.4.3   Low flow anaesthesia

Low flow anaesthesia, with semi-closed rebreathing systems but with a greater proportion of excess gas volume, should be possible with all appropriately maintained machines, even those of the older generation and conventional technical design. For the majority of machines, this fresh gas flow corresponds to the range of operation quoted by the manufacturers. The tolerances specified for testing leakproofness during technical inspection and maintenance generally meet the relevant requirements. Continuous measurement of the inspired oxygen concentration, the airway pressure and the minute volume with adjustable alarm limits are indispensable monitoring requirements to guarantee patient safety during the performance of any anaesthetic technique with low fresh gas flow.

7.5   References

1. CEN: Comit Europen de Normalisation. Anaesthetic Workstations and their Modules – Essential Requirements. prEN 740, Revision 6.0, 1994
2. Deutsches Institut für Normung: Deutsche Norm Inhalationsnarkosegeräte. Entwurf DIN 13 252 A1, Beuth, Belin (1991)
3. International Organization for Standardization. *ISO 5358 – Anaesthetic Machines for Use with Humans*, 2nd edn, 1992-01-15, ISO, Geneva (1992)

4. American Society for Testing and Materials:
   - ASTM designation: F 1161-88: Standard Specification for Minimum Performance and Safety Requirements for Components and Systems of Anesthesia Gas Machines. ASTM Standards (1988), pp. 509–532
   - ASTM designation: F 1280-89: Standard Specification for Minimum Performance and Safety Requirements for Anesthesia Breathing Systems. ASTM Standards (1989), pp. 560–571
   - ASTM designation: F 1101-90: Standard Specification for Ventilators Intended for Use During Anesthesia. ASTM Standards (1990), pp. 449–459
5. Baum, J. Technische Voraussetzungen für die Narkoseführung mit reduziertem Frischgasfluß. In *Alternative Methoden der Anästhesie* (eds P. Lawin, H. van Aken and U. Schneider) INA-Schriftenreihe, Bd. 50, Thieme, Stuttgart (1985), pp. 43–48
6. Droh, R. Practical application of the closed-circuit system. In *Closed-Circuit System and Other Innovations in Anaesthesia* (eds R. Droh and R. Spintge), Springer, Berlin (1986), pp. 8–12
7. Götz, H. and Obermayer, A. Wie zuverlässig ist die Narkosegasmessung bei niedrigem Frischgasflow? In *Narkosebeatmung: Low Flow, Minimal Flow, Geschlossenes System* (J.-P. A. H. Jantzen and P. P. Kleemann), Schattauer, Stuttgart (1989), pp. 77–87
8. von dem Hagen, T. and Kleinschmidt, L. Principles of low flow measurement for closed-circuit systems. In *Anaesthesia – Innovations in Management* (eds R. Droh, W. Erdmann and R. Spintge), Springer, Berlin (1985), pp. 10–15
9. Saunders, R. J., Calkins, J. M. and Goodin, T. G. Accuracy of rotameters and linear flowmeters. *Anesthesiology* **55** (Suppl.) A116 (1981)
10. Rügheimer, E. Low-flow und Closed-Circuit anaesthesia. In *Kombinationsanästhesie* (ed. W. Dick), Springer, Berlin (1985), pp. 116–135
11. Frankenberger, H. and Wallroth, C. F. Technische Konzeptionen für ein geschlossenes Narkosesystem. In *Geschlossenes System für Inhalationsnarkosen*, Internationales Symposium, Düsseldorf, 7–8 May 1982 (Abstract)
12. Cicman, J., Himmelwright, H., Skibo, V. and Yoder, J. *Operating Principles of Narkomed Anesthesia Systems*, North American Dräger, Telford (1993)
13. Siemens-Elema AB: Instructions for Use
    - Servo Anesthesia System (Servo Anesthesia Circle 985)
    - Siemens Vaporizer 950-952, Siemens-Elema AB, Solna
14. Frankenberger, H., Seidel, P. and Eichler, J. Optimierung eines Narkosemittelverdunsters für die Inhalationsnarkose. Jahrestagung der DGAW, Lübeck-Travemünde, 7.-8-Oktober 1976, Drägerwerk AG, Lübeck (1976)
15. Drägerwerk AG – Instructions for Use:
    - Anästhesie-Ventilator AV 1. GA 5162 (May 1989)
    - Cicero, Integrierter Narkose-Arbeitsplatz. GA 5131.001 (July 1991)
    - Cicero EM, Integrierter Narkose-Arbeitsplatz, GA 5131.100 d (Nov. 1993)
    - Kreissytem 8 ISO. GA 5371 (Sept. 1989)
    - Ergänzung 'Geschlossenes System' zur Gebrauchsanweisung 5371 Kreissystem 8 ISO (Oct. 1989)
    - Narkosemittelverdampfer Vapor 19. GA 5327.0 (Jan. 1983)
    - Narkosemittelverdampfer Vapor 19.n. GA 5327.0 (April 1986)
    - Narkosemittelverdampfer Vapor 19.n. GA 5327.0 (March 1991)
    - Narkosespiromat 650. GA 5161 (Oct. 1972)
    - Narkosespiromat 656. GA 5161.1 (June 1985)
    - Pulmomat 19 (19.1, 19.3). GA 5323 (June 1977)
    - SA 2/RA 2 Inhalation Anaesthetic Machine, GA 5152 e (Nov. 1992)
    - Sulla 808 M/V/MV, Inhalationsnarkosegerät. GA 5191.3 (Oct. 1989)
    - Möglichkeit zur Dosierung kleiner Frischgasmengen. Beilage zu den Gebrauchsanweisungen Sulla 808 (GA 5191.3) und Sulla 808 V-D (GA 5191.31) (May 1988)
    - Ventilog und Ventilog 2, Narkosebeatmungsgeräte. GA 5324.0 (March 1990)
    - Ventilog 3, Narkosebeatmungsgerät, GA 5324.100 d, Drägerwerk AG, Lübeck (June 1992)

16. Züchner, K., Raffauf, E. M. and Sonntag, H. Genauigkeit von Halothanverdampfern unter praxisnahen Betriebsbedingungen. *Anaesthesist*, **32** (Suppl.), 174 (1983)

17. Gilly, H. Zur Brauchbarkeit herkömmlicher Verdampfer bei Minimal flow. In *Narkosebeatmung: Low Flow, Minimal Flow, Geschlossenes System* (eds J.-P. A. H. Jantzen and P. P. Kleemann), Schattauer, Stuttgart (1989), pp. 67–76

18. Davey, A., Moyle, J. T. B. and Ward, C. S. *Ward's Anaesthetic Equipment*, 3rd edn, W. B. Saunders, London (1992)

19. Hill, D. W. and Lowe, H. J. Comparison of concentration of halothane in closed and semiclosed circuits during controlled ventilation. *Anesthesiology*, **23**, 291–298 (1962)

20. Gambro Engström AB: Engström Elsa Anesthesia System, User's Instructions, Gambro Engström AB, Bromma, Sweden (1988)

21. Rathgeber, J. *Praxis der maschinellen Beatmung*, MCN-Verlag, Nürnberg (1990)

22. Frankenberger, H. Techniche di Vaporizzazione: In *Anestesia a Bassi Flussi e a Circuito Chiuso* (ed. F. Giunta), Piccin Nuova Libraria, Padova (1992), pp. 97–115

23. Sticher, J., Müller, M., Zeidler, D., Jung, H.-J. and Hempelmann, G. Unbeabsichtigte Narkosegasüberdosierung bei den Narkoserespiratoren Servo 900 C und D. *Anästhesiol. Intensivmed. Notfallmed. Schmerzther.*, **29**, 163–164 (1994)

24. Versichelen, L. and Rolly, G. Mass-spectrometric evaluation of some recently introduced low flow, closed circuit systems. *Acta Anaesth. Belg.*, **41**, 225–237 (1990)

25. Deutsches Institut für Normung: Deutsche Norm Inhalationsnarkosegeräte. DIN 13 252, Beuth, Berlin (1984)

26. Graham, S. G. The desflurane Tec 6 vaporizer. *Br. J. Anaesth.* **72**, 470–473 (1994)

27. Hargasser, S., Hipp, R., Breinbauer, B., Mielke, L., Entholzner, E. and Rust, M. A lower solubility recommends the use of desflurane more than isoflurane, halothane, and enflurane under low-flow conditions. *J. Clin. Anesth.*, **7**, 49–53 (1995)

28. Weiskopf, R. B., Sampson, D. and Moore, M. A. The desflurane (Tec 6) vaporizer: design, design considerations and performance evaluation. *Br. J. Anaesth.*, **72**, 474–479 (1994)

29. Lockwood, G. G., Kadim, M. Y., Chakrabarty, M. K. and Whitwam, J. G. Clinical use of small soda lime canister in a low-flow to-and-fro system. *Anaesthesia*, **47**, 568–573 (1992)

30. Megamed AG: Gebrauchsanweisung Megamed 700. Version AH007, 02/89. Megamed AG, Cham (1989)

31. Leuenberger, M., Feigenwinter, P. and Zbinden, A. M. Gas leakage in eight anaesthesia circle systems. *Eur. J. Anaesthesiol.*, **9**, 121–127 (1992)

32. Amt Für Arbeitsschutz: Merkblatt für den Umgang mit Narkosegasen. Hansestadt Hamburg, August 1990, p. 8

33. Spintge, R. and Droh, R. The absolutely tight circuit system and the problem of excess humidity. *Anaesthesia – Innovations in Management* (eds R. Droh, W. Erdmann and R. Spintge), Springer, Berlin (1985), pp. 44–45

34. Baum, J. Clinical applications of low flow and closed circuit anaesthesia. *Acta Anaesth. Belg.*, **41**, 239–247 (1990)

35. Oeking, R. and K. H. Weis, K. H. Zur Sauerstoffkonzentration im Narkosekreissystem. II. Mitteilung: Abhängigkeit vom Typ des Kreissystems. *Anaesthesist*, **22**, 202–206 (1973)

36. Zbinden, A. M., Feigenwinter, P. and Hutmacher, M. Fresh gas utilisation of eight circle systems. *Br. J. Anaesth.*, **67**, 492–499 (1991)

37. Barth, L. and Meyer, M. CO_2-Absorption. In *Moderne Narkose*, Fischer, Stuttgart (1965), pp. 193–209

38. Gootjes, P. and Lagerweij, E. Quality comparison of different CO_2 absorbents. *Anaesthesist*, **30** 261–264 (1981)

39. Paravicini, D., Henning, K. and Vietor, G. Vergleichende Untersuchungen von verschiedenen Atemkalksorten. *Anästh. Intensivther. Notfallmed.*, **17**, 98–101 (1982)

40. Wulf, R., Siegel, E. and Wezurek, H. Drägersorb 800: Der Indikator-Atemkalk in Pillenform. *Medizintechnik aktuell*, **1**, 10–14 (1991)

41. Baum, J., Enzenauer, J., Krausse, Th. and Sachs, G. Atemkalk – Nutzungsdauer, Verbrauch und Kosten in Abhängigkeit vom Frischgasfluß. *Anaesthesiol. Reanimat.*, **18**, 108–113 (1993)

42. Oehmig, H. Atemkalk '85/'86. *Anästh. Intensivmed.*, **27**, 397–399 (1986)

43. Lotz, P., Siegel, E. and Spilker, D. *Grundbegriffe der Beatmung*, GIT Verlag Ernst Giebeler, Darmstadt (1984)
44. Klement, W. and Stühmeier, K. Gefahren bei Beatmungsgeräten ohne Reservoir schon bei mittlerem Frischgasflow? *Anaesthesist*, **38** (Suppl. 1), 126 (1989)
45. Baum, J. and Schneider, U. Die Brauchbarkeit verschiedener Narkosebeatmungsgeräte für die Minimal-Flow-Anästhesie. *Anästh. Intensivmed.*, **24**, 263–269 (1983)
46. Spieß, W. Narkose im geschlossenen System mit kontinuierlicher inspiratorischer Sauerstoffmessung. *Anaesthesist*, **26**, 503–513 (1977)
47. Aldrete, J. A., Adolph, A. J., Hanna, L. M., Farag, A. and Ghaemmaghami, M. Fresh gas flow rate and I:E ratio affect tidal volume in anaesthesia ventilators. In *Quantitative Anaesthesia* (eds K. Ackern, H. Frankenberger, E. Konecny and K. Steinbereithner), Anaesthesiology and Intensive Care Medicine, Vol. 204. Springer, Berlin (1989), pp. 72–80
48. Baum, J. and Sachs, G. Frischgasflow und Narkosebeatmung – Technische Voraussetzungen für die adäquate Nutzung von Rückatemsystemen. *Anästh. Intensivther. Notfallmed.*, **25**, 72–78 (1990)
49. Bund, M. and Kirchner, E. Respiratorbedingte Veränderungen der Beatmungsparameter bei Reduktion des Frischgasflusses. *Anästh. Intensivmed.*, **32**, 179–183 (1991)
50. Lowe, H. J. and Ernst, E. A. *Quantitative Practice of Anesthesia*, Williams and Wilkins, Baltimore (1981)
51. Carl Heyer Medizintechnologie: Technical Data DOGMA, 1/93. Carl-Heyer-Straße 1/3, 56130 Bad Ems (1993)
52. Schepp, R. M., Erdmann, W., Westerkamp, B. and Faithful, N. S. Automatic ventilation during closed circuit anaesthesia. In: *Anaesthesia – Innovations in Management* (eds R. Droh, W. Erdmann and R. Spintge), Springer, Berlin (1985), pp. 48–53
53. Spain, J. A., Jannett, T. C. and Ernst, E. A. The Alabama automated closed-circuit anesthesia project. In *Future Anesthesia Delivery Systems* (eds B. R. Brown, J. L. Calkins and R. J. Saunders), F. A. Davies, Philadelphia (1984), pp. 177–183
54. Westenskow, D. R., Jordan, W. S. and Gehmlich, D. S. Electronic feedback control and measurement of oxygen consumption during closed circuit anaesthesia. In *Low Flow and Closed System Anesthesia* (eds J. A. Aldrete, H. J. Lowe and R. W. Virtue), Grune and Stratton, New York (1979), pp. 135–146
55. Westenskow, D. R. and Wallroth, C. F. Closed-loop control for anesthesia breathing systems. *J. Clin. Monit*, **6**, 249–256 (1990)
56. Physio, B. V. PhysioFlex, Gesloten Anaesthesie Ventilator. Physio Medical Systems, Hoofddorp (1990)

Monitoring

8.1 Technical regulations: safety facilities for inhalation anaesthetic machines

The comments on monitoring will deal primarily with the monitoring of the gas composition in the breathing system. Here, at this interface between patient and anaesthetic machine[1], changes, determined essentially by the fresh gas composition and the patient's uptake, can be observed. While with high flow, the gas composition within the breathing system can be estimated easily from the composition of the fresh gas, this becomes more difficult with lower fresh gas flows[2]. That is why the question arises as to whether additional monitoring devices are required to guarantee patient safety during the performance of low flow anaesthesia.

Independent of the fresh gas flow selection, routine monitoring of the patient and the performance of the machine is obligatory and provided by respective technical regulations, recommendations of scientific and professional organizations and relevant teachings[3–12]. Among other issues, they comprise permanent clinical observation of the electrocardiogram, regular checks on circulation, measurement of the airway pressure and the expired tidal or minute volume (Table 8.1).

According to regulations in different European countries and in the USA, continuous monitoring of the inspired oxygen concentration[3,5,7] and, in Germany since 1991, even monitoring of the anaesthetic agent concentration are mandatory[7]. Monitoring of the anaesthetic agent concentration is also laid down in the draft of the common European norm as an obligatory safety standard for inhalation anaesthetic machines[5]. In addition, continuous monitoring of the expired carbon dioxide concentration will be required. Thus, comprehensive monitoring of the anaesthetic gas composition will be mandatory, as it is already provided for in the modern generation of anaesthetic workstations.

8.2 Main- and side-stream gas analysers

The analysis of gas concentrations by locating the sensor directly in the breathing or patient hose system is referred to as main-stream measurement (Figure 8.1a,b). The advantage of this method is that gas concentrations are

Table 8.1   Safety facilities of inhalation anaesthetic machines

SAFETY FACILITIES				
Oxygen shortage signal	A*	B		D	
Nitrous oxide cut-off	A	B		D	
Oxygen ratio controller		B		D	
MONITORING OF EQUIPMENT FUNCTION					
Airway pressure with disconnection and obstruction alarm	A	B		D	E
Expired gas volume	A	B	C	D	E
Inspired oxygen concentration	A	B	C	D	E
Volatile anaesthetic concentration	A	B	C	D	E
Carbon dioxide concentration		B	C	D	
MONITORING OF PHYSIOLOGICAL PARAMETERS					
Stethoscope			C	D	
ECG			C	D	
Blood pressure measurement			C	D	
Temperature measurement			C	D	
Pulse oximetry			C	D	

*A, Conforms to German DIN 13252 and MedGV[6,7].
B, Draft of the new common European norm prEN 740[5].
C, Recommendations on standard monitoring by Whitcher et al.[11].
D, Guidelines by DGAI (German Association for Anaesthesia and Intentive Care Medicine) and BDA (Professional Organisation of Anaesthetists)[4].
E, Special recommendations on monitoring for safe performance of anaesthesia with a fresh gas flow equal or less than 1 l/min[11,13-16].

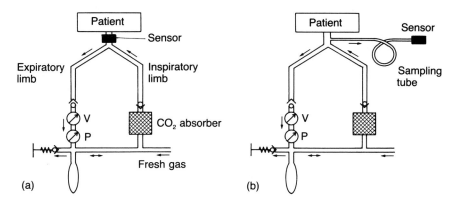

Figure 8.1   Position of sensors for measurement of gas concentrations: (a) measurement directly in the gas stream = main-stream measurement; (b) measurement by withdrawing sampling gas out of the system = side-stream measurement (From Pockrand[17], by permission)

measured directly in the breathing gas stream, and may be displayed without any significant delay if the electronic response time of the device is correspondingly low. However, placement of the sensor directly on to the tube connector is rather involved in daily clinical routine. Due to hygiene regulations, parts of the sensor contaminated by the exhaled gas have to be replaced with each patient, or single use bacterial filters have to be used. In addition, the weight of the main-stream sensor is liable to displace the tube, whereby the free passage of breathing gas may be impaired.

For measurement with the side-stream technique, the gas sample is sucked out of the breathing system and passed to a separate measuring device via a tube. In general, the sample is taken from a point between the tube connector and the Y-piece of the patient hose system. The simple technique can generally be undertaken without any problems during daily clinical practice.

It must be considered on the other hand that, depending on the sampling flow and the dimensions of the sampling hose, alterations of the gas concentrations in the system may be indicated at the display of the monitor only after a certain time delay. In addition, the amplitude and the characteristics of the measured signal may be subjected to considerable changes by the passage of sampling gas through the hose[17,18].

8.2.1   Return of sampling gas

When a side-stream measuring device is used during low flow anaesthesia, the sampling gas should be returned into the expiratory limb of the breathing system after the measuring procedure is completed. Otherwise, the loss of sampling gas may result in a volume shortage in the system, especially if the sampling gas flow is higher than 100 ml/min and the fresh gas flow about 500 ml/min. If conventional 8 or 9 ISO circle absorber systems (Drägerwerk, Lübeck, Germany) are used, this can be accomplished by using a special self-sealing quick connector normally used for airway pressure measurement. A 30 μm bacterial filter should be connected into the gas return tube to preclude contamination. Within the range of normal airway pressure, the change in pressure at the sampling gas outlet resulting from controlled ventilation has very little influence on the measurement. But even so, some gas analysers are fitted with pressure compensation; for example, the Datex monitors (Datex, Helsinki, Finland) or the PM 8020 and 8050 monitors (Drägerwerk, Lübeck, Germany).

Another aspect needs to be considered if sampling gas is returned into the system. If the sampling gas is subject to a measuring technique which alters the molecular structure of the gas, for instance ultraviolet absorption or mass spectrometry, it is self-evident that this gas should not be returned into the breathing system.

Paramagnetic measurement of oxygen concentration calls for simultaneous reference measurement with a gas of known oxygen content. The multi-gas analyser Capnomac (Datex, Helsinki, Finland), for instance, works with a sampling gas flow of 200 ml/min and, in addition, needs approximately 30 ml/min ambient air as reference gas. Having passed the measurement device, both the sampling and the reference gas are returned together into the breathing system. Using extremely low fresh gas flows, this additional supply of ambient air into the system results in a slow accumulation of nitrogen.

Accumulation of nitrogen within the breathing system can also be observed with low flow anaesthesia if the measuring system is intermittently calibrated with ambient air. The Dräger monitors 8020 and 8050 (Drägerwerk, Lübeck, Germany), for instance, are calibrated with ambient air every 5–10 min

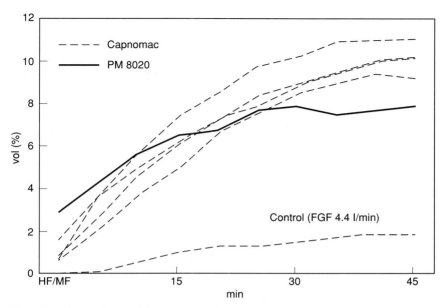

Figure 8.2 Accumulation of foreign gases (nitrogen, water vapour and trace gases) during performance of minimal flow anaesthesia with return of sampled gas. HF/MF, time of flow reduction. Measurements performed with a Capnomac gas analyser (Datex, Helsinki, Finland) on different patient collectives with the AV 1, Elsa, Megamed 700 and Sulla 800 anaesthetic machines. The measurement with the PM 8020 gas analyser (Drägerwerk, Lübeck, Germany) was performed at the Cicero anaesthetic workstation. Note: In the control group the high fresh gas flow is maintained during the whole course of anaesthesia

during the first 30 min, and thereafter every 30 min at a rate of 150 ml/min (Figure 8.2).

The present author cannot agree totally with the recommendation of Bengtson et al.[19], not to return the sampling gas to the breathing system during low flow anaesthesia, in order to avoid nitrogen accumulation. Whereas this recommendation may be acceptable in low flow anaesthesia, in which an excess gas volume of about 600 ml/min is used, in minimal flow anaesthesia the additional loss of the sampling gas into the scavenging system will result in gas deficiency within the breathing system and corresponding alterations of ventilatory patterns. If nitrogen accumulation results in a significant change of the anaesthetic gas composition, a short wash-out phase using high fresh gas flow over a period of about 5 min should be carried out. A sampling gas return tube is already a technical feature of some modern anaesthetic machines such as the Cicero EM (Drägerwerk, Lübeck, Germany).

8.3   Measurement of oxygen concentration

If low flow anaesthesia is performed, it has to be considered that the lower the fresh gas flow, the greater will be the difference between its oxygen concentration and the concentration of oxygen within the breathing system (see Section 3.1). Furthermore, it must be borne in mind that, with the increase of the rebreathing gas volume, the inspired oxygen concentration is determined to a considerably greater extent by the patient's individual oxygen consumption than in high flow anaesthesia. These are the reasons why continuous monitoring of oxygen concentration in the breathing system is indispensable to ensure patient safety if anaesthesia is performed with low fresh gas flow[20].

All the various methods of oxygen concentration measurement may be applied. Electrochemical techniques with a response time between 5 and 20 s are essentially slower than paramagnetic, magneto-acoustic or mass spectrometric measurement with a response time between 100 and 450 ms. But extended response times do not impair safety in any way, since concentration changes in the breathing system with low flow anaesthesia proceed with considerable time delay. Electrochemical methods of oxygen concentration measurement may be affected by humidity, but this problem can be solved by means of humidity condensors. The measuring accuracy of 1–2% by volume, which is unanimously quoted for all the different methods, is quite adequate to satisfy clinical requirements.

Measuring techniques which are based on the paramagnetic properties of oxygen molecules work with such a fast response time that the measured signal can be resolved into the inspired and expired values. By the additional measurement of expired oxygen concentration, it is possible to evaluate the efficiency of nitrogen wash-out during preoxygenation and to recognize early the development of hypoxia caused by hypoventilation during the emergence phase. Nevertheless, the expired oxygen concentration is not a reliable parameter for evaluating the oxygen consumption, since it is determined to a large extent by the actual nitrous oxide uptake. This is why, following

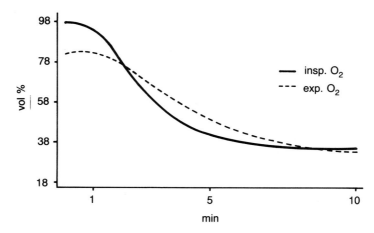

Figure 8.3 Inspired and expired oxygen concentrations during wash-in of nitrous oxide–oxygen mixture (32% O_2, 68% N_2O) after sufficient preoxygenation. During the first 10 min the expired oxygen concentration is higher than the inspired due to the initial high nitrous oxide uptake

adequate denitrogenation with pure oxygen, the admixture of nitrous oxide results in the following phenomenon: because of the initially high nitrous oxide uptake, the expired oxygen concentration is higher than the inspired. It takes a period of about 20 min of normoventilation to attain the physiological inspired–expired oxygen difference of 4.5%. (Figure 8.3). With a view to patient safety, continuous monitoring of inspired oxygen concentration alone can be regarded as appropriate. In the particular case of anaesthesia with very low fresh gas flow, a reduction in the expired oxygen concentration can clearly be recognized from the distinct simultaneous decrease of the inspired oxygen concentration (see Section 3.1).

Finally, it is emphasized again that continuous monitoring of oxygen concentration is an absolute necessity during anaesthesia with reduced fresh gas flows. This is already provided by the standards of several countries, which demand all inhalational anaesthesia machines to be equipped with this safety device.

8.4   Measurement of volatile anaesthetic concentration

The concentration of inhalational anaesthetics can be measured by way of mass spectrometry, crystal oscillometry, infrared absorption, photoacoustic and Raman spectrometry[16,18,21,22]. All these different approaches are employed in clinical practice, but photoacoustic spectrometry and infrared absorption have become the standard clinical methods. Interference by nitrous oxide, carbon dioxide and water vapour can readily be compensated for, and the accuracy of $\pm 0.15\%$ by volume which is quoted for the majority of measurement devices is completely acceptable for clinical use[15]. However, crystal oscillometry in the main stream (EMMA, Engström, Bromma, Sweden) has not proved to be satisfactory because of its great sensitivity with respect to humidity[23,24]. Where the Servo Gas Monitor 120 (Siemens-Elema, Solna, Sweden) is concerned, a side-stream analyser using the same measurement technique, the cross-sensitivity to water vapour could be considerably reduced. With respect to drift and precision, this unit is also suitable for use in low flow anaesthesia.

The difference between the anaesthetic concentration in the fresh gas and that in the breathing system increases with reduction of the fresh flow (see Section 3.3.2). With extremely low fresh gas flows, repeated change of anaesthetic fresh gas concentration and repeated flow variation, it is virtually impossible, even for an anaesthetist experienced in low flow techniques, to estimate precisely the anaesthetic concentration in the breathing system. On the other hand, even drastic changes of the anaesthetic concentration in the fresh gas cause only extremely slow changes in the breathing system gas composition, which can be attributed to the long time constant in low flow anaesthesia. Thus, the risk of accidental over- or underdosage of inhalational anaesthetic is distinctly lower than with high flow anaesthesia. Anaesthesia with low fresh gas flow in particular allows for an ample period of time to adjust the depth of anaesthesia according to the clinical state of the patient.

An obvious safety problem is encountered in making a change from low to high fresh gas flow. With low fresh gas flow, considerably higher concentrations of volatile anaesthetic in the fresh gas are used than with high fresh gas flow. In changing from low to high flow, the fresh gas concentration of the volatile anaesthetic has to be reduced and thus adapted to the modified flow, since otherwise the concentration of the anaesthetic in the system will increase drastically in only a short time. On the other hand, there is the risk of underdosage if the concentration of the inhalational anaesthetic is not appropriately increased in the case of a reduction of fresh gas flow. Accidental incorrect dosage resulting from changes in the fresh gas flow can only be detected sufficiently early if the anaesthetic concentration in the breathing system is measured and monitored continuously[14,25].

The use of a vaporizer inside the circle (VIC) has always been proscribed for positive pressure ventilation on account of the potential for drastic rises in vapour concentration. The advent of agent analysers invites the reappraisal of this technique, but it must be accepted that the monitor has to be considered part of the dosing system itself. The same statement holds for the use of a single analyser during direct injection of liquid agent. This is acknowledged by the inclusion of a 'guardian unit' in the PhysioFlex anaesthetic machine as a safety back-up device.

8.4.1   Should anaesthetic agent measurement be performed in the fresh gas or in the breathing system?

There are two alternatives for monitoring inhalational anaesthetics: either the anaesthetic concentration in the breathing system or its fresh gas concentration can be measured. Monitoring the anaesthetic concentration in the breathing system[14] is the only way of precluding false dosage resulting from machine malfunction or handling errors. Measuring in the fresh gas will definitely afford less safety, since only the vaporizer function and adjustment are monitored but not the actual dosage of the inhalational anaesthetic. After all, the technical component by means of which inhalational anaesthetics are really dosed is actually the breathing system. This is where the anaesthetic mixture supplied to the patient is composed in a complex process, determined by the technical design and functional state of the breathing system, the fresh gas flow and the uptake.

The resultant safety problem can be explained by an example. A 75 kg patient is anaesthetized with isoflurane via a rebreathing system, whereby the isoflurane concentration is continuously and simultaneously measured and monitored in the fresh gas as well as in the inspiratory limb of the breathing system. At the beginning of anaesthesia, the upper alarm limit of both systems is set to 2% (Figure 8.4).

With a fresh gas flow of 4.4 l/min, the isoflurane concentration is initially set to 1.5%. After 15 min, the flow is reduced to 0.5 l/min, while at the same time the anaesthetic concentration is increased to 2.5% (A). After a period of 30 min, the clinical situation calls for a deeper level of anaesthesia, so that the fresh gas isoflurane concentration is increased to 5% but the flow is left unchanged (B). Due to the long time constant of the system, the changes of the inspired isoflurane concentration proceed very slowly and moderately. The upper alarm limit of 2.0% of the device monitoring the agent concentration in the breathing system can be maintained independent of the fresh gas flow selected. On the other hand, the alarm limit of the device monitoring the fresh gas concentration has to be adjusted according to the

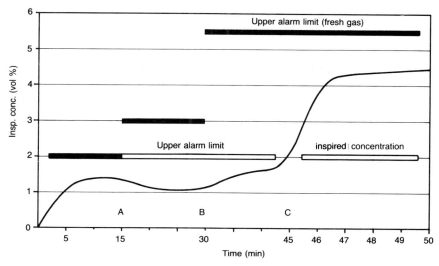

Figure 8.4   Simultaneous monitoring of volatile anaesthetic concentration in the fresh gas and in the breathing system. Only if the concentration within the breathing system is measured will it be possible to adjust the alarm limits independently of the fresh gas flow. Only application of this technique will ensure reliable detection of accidental overdose. (Curve, inspired isoflurane concentration; bars, adjustment of the upper alarm limits) (From Baum[14])

newly set fresh gas concentration. This means that at flow reduction it has to be increased to 3.0% (A) and at point B to as high as 5.5%.

Emergence from anaesthesia is induced after 45 min by increasing the fresh gas flow to 4.0 l/min (C). Assume that the vaporizer is accidentally left at a setting of 5%. The resulting rapid increase of the inspired anaesthetic concentration to almost 5.0% will only be recognized by continuous monitoring of the inspired concentration. On the other hand, the device monitoring the fresh gas concentration will not warn of the danger of overdosage. This example demonstrates convincingly that only by monitoring the anaesthetic concentration in the breathing system can comprehensive protection against misdosage be achieved. Only if this technique is adopted can the alarm limits be adjusted independently of the fresh gas flow.

As most anaesthetic incidents are based on inappropriate human behaviour and decisions, and not on actual malfunction of machines[26,27], misdosage resulting from handling errors must be detected by the monitoring techniques employed. And last but not least, only continuous measurement of the anaesthetic agent concentration in the breathing system facilitates safe and judicious performance of low flow anaesthesia[25].

8.5   Measurement of nitrous oxide concentration

The question whether the concentration of nitrous oxide should also be monitored continuously is still under discussion. It is obvious that an overdose of nitrous oxide is precluded by continuous monitoring of the inspired oxygen concentration. Therefore, additional measurement of nitrous oxide concentration seems to be unnecessary. However, misdosage of nitrous oxide cannot always be reliably detected by merely measuring the oxygen concentration. In some anaesthetic machines, entrance of ambient air is effected via a special ambient air valve. In case of gas volume shortage in the breathing system, the opening of this safety valve prevents possible alterations of the ventilatory patterns. This is to ensure adequate ventilation of the patient in spite of inadequate fresh gas supply. A case of considerable misdosage of nitrous oxide was observed during the use of a Megamed 700 machine (Figure 8.5). The depicted drastic decrease in nitrous oxide concentration resulted from the entrance of ambient air into the breathing system via an ambient air valve. That was due to inadequate adjustment of the excess gas discharge valve to the fresh gas flow. In this case, nitrous oxide misdosage could only be detected by continuous nitrous oxide monitoring, as the inspired oxygen concentration remained absolutely stable.

In addition, the accumulation of foreign gas, which may be observed in low flow anaesthesia (see Figure 8.2), can only be assessed by additional measurement of the nitrous oxide concentration[16,25]. The proportion of foreign gas can then be calculated from the deficit of the sum of all measured inspired gas concentrations (oxygen, nitrous oxide, inhalational anaesthetic). The concent of water vapour in the inspired gas which, depending on the gas temperature ranges between 2.3% and 4%, is ignored in this calculation. During performance of long-term anaesthesia with extremely low fresh gas flows and return of the sampling gas (see Section 8.2.1), the proportion of foreign gas is liable to rise to values greater than 15%. If the nitrous oxide concentration is too low, due to the admixture of foreign gases, the system

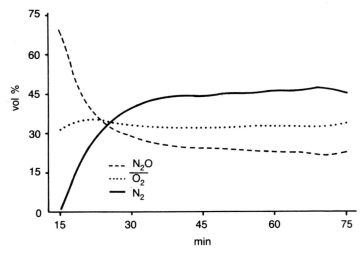

Figure 8.5   Entrainment of room air into the breathing system via an ambient air safety valve during minimal flow anaesthesia due to inappropriate adjustment of the excess gas discharge valve (Megamed 700 anaesthetic machine, Megamed, Cham, Switzerland). In the depicted case, this error in operating the machine can only be detected by means of nitrous oxide concentration measurement, as the oxygen concentration remains stable (Patient aged 60 years, weight 68 kg, height 1.60 m)

may be flushed for 2–5 min with a high fresh gas flow. This procedure eliminates the foreign gas from the breathing system and the nitrous oxide concentration can be re-established at the nominal value.

8.6   Measurement of carbon dioxide concentration

In clinical practice, the infrared absorption technique is mainly used for the measurement of carbon dioxide concentration. Both main-stream and side-stream analysers are available. Both capnometry and capnography add considerably to the improvement of patient safety, since this parameter provides considerable information about the patient and the anaesthetic machine[28]. However, every alteration of this complex information needs careful and comprehensive analysis[29]. It is self-evident that this analysis also requires detailed knowledge of possible flow-specific artefacts.

8.6.1   Flow-specific artefacts of the capnogram

If sampling gas which is taken out of the patient hose system at the Y-piece is analysed, the reduction of the fresh gas flow is liable to cause contamination of the expired gas with inspiratory gas. This phenomenon may be observed if controlled ventilation is performed with conventional anaesthetic machines featuring constant flow of fresh gas into the system and hanging bellows, which are actively expanded during expiration[28,30]. With both main- and side-stream measurement, the capnographic curves do not show the typical waveform with a slightly ascending expiratory plateau. On the contrary, the curves tend to descend during the course of exhalation without having formed a distinct plateau. Mostly the capnographic curves have superimposed cardiogenic oscillations (Figure 8.6). These artificial changes of the capnograms result from the fact that the reduction of the fresh gas flow results in

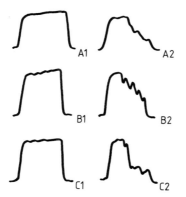

Figure 8.6   Artificial changes in configuration of capnographic curves due to fresh gas flow reduction: with high flow of 4.4 l/min, typical waveform with ascending plateau (A1, B1, C1); after flow reduction to 0.5 l/min, descending curve during exhalation without a plateau (A2, B2, C2). Records taken during the use of a conventional anaesthetic machine with continuous supply of fresh gas into the breathing system and hanging bellows

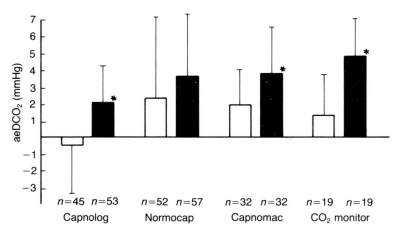

Figure 8.7   Increase of the arterial–end-expired carbon dioxide partial pressure difference (aeDCO$_2$) due to changing from high to low fresh gas flow. Identical changes of readings in both, main-stream (Capnolog) and side-stream monitors (Normocap, Capnomac, CO$_2$ monitor). White columns, aeDCO$_2$ with high fresh gas flow (4.2–4.4 l/min); black columns, aeDCO$_2$ with low fresh gas flow (0.5 l/min) (*Statistical significance of difference (Student's t-test): $p < 0.001$)

an increase of initial negative expiratory pressure with corresponding changes in the gas flow at the Y-piece. The changes may be accentuated by a high sampling gas flow in case of side-stream anaesthetic gas measurement.

Correspondingly, the arterial–end-expired partial pressure difference of carbon dioxide (aeDCO$_2$) increases in both, side- and main-stream measurement. The aeDCO$_2$ is the difference between the arterial carbon dioxide partial pressure (PaCO$_2$), obtained by blood gas analysis, and the end-expiratory carbon dioxide partial pressure (PeCO$_2$), calculated from the expired carbon dioxide concentration. In patients who are not suffering from pulmonary disease, this value increases by about 3 mmHg (Figure 8.7). The aeDCO$_2$ is a measure of the alveolar dead space ventilation which, under normal physiological conditions, amounts to about 4 mmHg[31]. In a considerably number of diseases causing imbalances of the lung's ventilation perfusion ratio[31,32], this value is increased, which also applies if gas free from carbon dioxide is admixed to the expired gas[33,34]. On the contrary, the aeDCO$_2$ decreases with forced ventilation[31]. If, during performance of low flow anaesthesia, a defined arterial carbon dioxide partial pressure is adjusted precisely by capnometry, the PaCO$_2$ should be established by blood gas analysis only if the flow has already been reduced. The PeCO$_2$ should be measured at the same time and the aeDCO$_2$, specific to the low flow condition, can then be calculated from these two values. This is the only way of estimating an actual PaCO$_2$ correctly during the following course of anaesthesia by using the formula:

$$P\text{a}CO_2 = P\text{e}CO_2 + \text{ae}DCO_2$$

The aforementioned procedure-specific alterations in carbon dioxide measurement are relevant for anaesthetic practice in so far as misinterpretations of capnometric values and capnogram configuration can only be prevented if these facts are known[28]. However, these artificial alterations of the carbon dioxide signal and resultant increase of $aeDCO_2$ are not observed if low flow anaesthesia is performed with anaesthetic machines of the new generation (see Chapter 7), featuring a gas reservoir and discontinuous fresh gas supply.

8.6.2 Zero calibration

Main-stream and side-stream analysers may differ greatly in respect of the technique of zero calibration. While in most side-stream analysers, zero calibration is effected by reference measurement with carbon dioxide free gas, in some of the main-stream analysers it is performed during the inspiratory phase. This calibration technique can only be correct under the

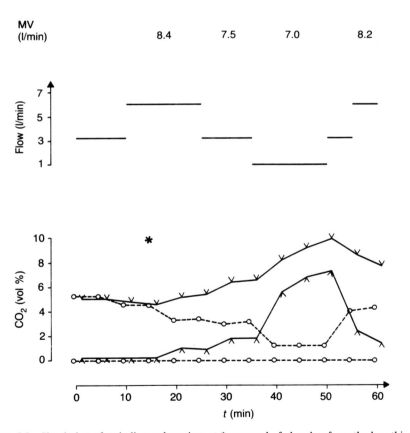

Figure 8.8 Simulation of soda lime exhaustion: at *, removal of absorber from the breathing system; ———, measurement with Normocap (side-stream analyser); – – –, measurement with Capnolog D (main-stream analyser). The inspired and expired carbon dioxide concentration increase excessively with reduction of the fresh gas flow, but decrease only with the increase of flow. However, the readings displayed by the Capnolog D are lower, the higher the inspired carbon dioxide concentration. Zero calibration is effected with inspired gas during each ventilation stroke (Patient aged 16 years, weight 70 kg, height 1.83 m)

proviso that the inspired gas is definitely free from carbon dioxide. If carbon dioxide absorption is insufficient due to soda lime exhaustion, this will not cause any serious problem with high fresh gas flows due to the low share of rebreathing volume and the resultant high wash-out effect[35]. But in the case of low flow anaesthesia, an excessive increase of the carbon dioxide concentration in the inspiratory limb of the breathing system will result from exhaustion of the absorbent. This equipment failure, which is especially serious with low flow anaesthesia, and which is not reliably indicated by a colour change of the indicator (see Section 7.2.5), cannot be detected by means of such main-stream analysers. On the contrary, these devices indicate paradoxically low figures in the event of soda lime exhaustion (Figure 8.8). Both expired and inspired carbon dioxide concentration can be reliably measured by means of side-stream analysers, in which the zero calibration is effected with carbon dioxide free reference gas, or by main-stream analysers, working with a chopper wheel and different filters. Only by these techniques of zero calibration it is possible to detect exhaustion of soda lime reliably, which is essential in low flow anaesthesia.

If, however, carbon dioxide absorption is ensured by using double 1-litre canisters or Jumbo absorbers, and if in addition the soda lime is regularly exchanged after each working day, monitoring of absorber function by continuous carbon dioxide measurement must not be assumed to be necessary for safe performance of low flow anaesthesia[2,36].

8.6.3 Implications for anaesthetic practice

With capnometry and capnography the anaesthetist has two monitoring parameters available, which, independent of the fresh gas flow selected, provide essential information on the clinical condition of the patient and the function of the anaesthetic machine[28]. This monitoring adds considerably to the safety of the anaesthetized patient[12,37]. It is the present author's view that it should be available at each anaesthetic workplace, irrespective of the anaesthetic technique applied. The forthcoming European norm will demand carbon dioxide monitoring as a standard safety device for all inhalation anaesthetic machines[5].

It is for these reasons of safety that in low flow anaesthesia only monitoring equipment which ensures reliable measurement of the carbon dioxide concentration should be used. Main-stream analysers whose zero point is calibrated by the use of inspired gas are not suitable for this anaesthetic technique. However, if continuous monitoring of inspired and expired carbon dioxide concentration is available, the soda lime should not be discarded as a routine measure, but should, for reasons of economy and ecology, be used until it is exhausted[36].

8.7   Multi-gas analysers

Complex analysis of gas composition in the breathing system is made possible by using a mass spectrometer or a multi-gas analyser. To date, only a few clinical centres are making significant use of mass spectrometry in routine anaesthetic practice[38–40].

However, several different multi-gas analysers are now available for clinical use. These devices either work on the principle of infrared absorption spectrometry (Datex, Dräger, Hellige, Nellcor), photoacoustic spectrometry (Brüel and Kjaer, Hewlett Packard) or Raman scattering (Ohmeda)[22]. All these different measurement techniques facilitate simultaneous measurement of carbon dioxide, nitrous oxide and volatile anaesthetic concentration. In some of these devices, oxygen concentration is determined by the paramagnetic technique. The extremely short response time permits measurement of the inspired and expired oxygen concentration. All these units are side-stream analysers which can be easily handled. They work reliably and are barely susceptible to malfunction, assisting the anaesthetist in analysing the gas composition in the system and its changes during the course of anaesthesia. The previously mentioned measurement techniques do not modify the gas molecules, so that the sampling gas can be returned to the breathing system once it has passed the device[17]. Accumulation of foreign gas has to be expected as, in addition to the sampling gas, gas for reference measurement and calibration routines is also drawn into the system. However, foreign gas accumulation takes place very slowly and can reliably be detected by the simultaneous measurement of oxygen and nitrous oxide. If required, this gas can be eliminated by briefly flushing the system with a high fresh gas flow.

Automatic gas identification is a great advantage in concentration measurement of volatile anaesthetics. Setting errors in devices without this

	Disconnection	Hypoventilation	Oesophageal intubation	Hypoxic gas mixture	Overdose by anaesthetics	Hypovolaemia	Pneumothorax	Air embolism	Hyperthermia	Aspiration	Arrhythmia	Acid-base disbalance	Overdose i.v. drug
Pulse oximetry	●	●	●	●			●	●	■	■	■		●
Capnometry	▲	●	▲			■	■	●	▲	■		●	■
Spirometry	▲	▲	■				■			■			■
Blood pressure					●	▲	■	●					●
Conc. of vol. anaesthetics	■				▲								
Insp. O₂ concentration				▲									
ECG						■					▲		
Temperature									●				
Auscultation	●	■	●			■	■	■		■	●		■

Figure 8.9 Value of different monitoring parameters for early detection of complications. ▲, Maximum value; ●, medium value; ■, low value (From Whitcher et al.[11], by permission)

facility may result in the display of wrong readings with clinically relevant deviation from real concentrations[15,41]. At present, there are only a few gas analysers which feature automatic gas identification.

Without doubt the use of multi-gas analysers will considerably increase the acceptance of adequate routine reduction of fresh gas flow. It facilitates the performance of the different techniques of low flow anaesthesia[13-16,18,21,25]. In addition, it has to be emphasized that the equipment for continuous monitoring of anaesthetic gas composition in the breathing system, which is required for safe performance of minimal flow anaesthesia, in accordance with the draft of the new common European norm will be an integral part of safety facilities of inhalation anaesthetic machines. Together with capnometry, continuous analysis of anaesthetic gas composition renders possible the comprehensive monitoring of both the patient's physical status and the functions of the anaesthetic machine, so that virtually all potential complications can be detected sufficiently early (Figure 8.9).

8.8   References

1. Frankenberger, H. Monitoring während Narkosen mit reduziertem Frischgasfluß. In *Alternative Methoden der Anästhesie* (eds P. Lawin, H. van Aken and U. Schneider), INA-Schriftenreihe, Bd. 50. Thieme, Stuttgart (1985), pp. 19–32
2. Nunn, J. F. Monitoring of totally closed systems. In *Low Flow and Closed System Anesthesia* (eds J. A. Aldrete, H. J. Lowe and R. W. Virtue), Grune and Stratton, New York (1979), pp. 199–209
3. American Society for Testing and Materials: ASTM designation: F 1161-88: Standard Specification for Minimum Performance and Safety Requirements for Components and Systems of Anesthesia Gas Machines. ASTM Standards (1988), pp. 509–532
4. Schmucker. P. Qualitätssicherung in der Anästhesiologie. Fortschreibung der Richtlinien der Deutschen Gesellschaft für Anästhesiologie und Intensivmedizin und des Berufsverbandes Deutscher Anästhesisten (*Anästh. Intensivmed.*, **30**, 307–314 (1989)). Anästh. Intensivmed. **36**, 250–254 (1995)
5. CEN: Comit Europen de Normalisation. *Anaesthetic Workstations and their Modules – Essential Requirements.* prEN 740, Revision 6.0, 1994
6. Deutsches Institut fur Normung: Deutsche Norm Inhalationsnarkosegeräte. DIN 13 252. Beuth, Berlin (1984)
7. Deutsches Institut für Normung: Deutsche Norm Inhalationsnarkosegeräte. Entwurf DIN 13 252 A1. Beuth, Berlin (1991)
8. International Organization for Standardization. *ISO 5358 – Anaesthetic Machines for Use with Humans*, 2nd edition, 1992-01-15, ISO, Geneva (1992)
9. Pasch, T. Die Überwachung des Patienten in der Narkose. *Anaesthesist*, **35**, 708–720 (1986)
10. Pasch, T. Basismonitoring: Empfehlungen und Standards. *Anaesthesist* **40** (Suppl. 2), S126 (1991)
11. Whitcher, C., Ream, A. K., Parsons, E. *et al.* Anesthetic mishaps and the cost of monitoring: a proposed standard for monitoring equipment. *J. Clin. Monit.*, **4**, 5–15 (1988)
12. Winter, A. and Spence, A. A. An international consensus on monitoring? *Br. J. Anaesth.*, **64**, 263–266 (1990)
13. Baum, J. Technische Voraussetzungen für die Narkoseführung mit reduziertem Frieschgasfluß. In *Alternative Methoden der Anästhesie* (eds P. Lawin, H. van Aken and U. Schneider), INA-Bd. 50, Thieme, Stuffgart (1985), pp. 43–48

14. Baum, J. Die Messung der Anästhesiemittelkonzentration. *Anästh. Intensivmed*, **32**, 284–286 (1991)
15. Gilly, H. Muß die Konzentration volatiler Anästhetika überwacht werden? *Anaesthesist*, **40** (Suppl. 2), (1991)
16. Jantzen, J.-P. A. H. Monitoring der Narkosebeatmung. In *Narkosebeatmung: Low Flow, Minimal Flow, Geschlossenes System* (eds J.-P. A. H. Jantzen, P. Schaffauer), Stuttgart (1989), pp. 25–47
17. Pockrand, I. Optische Gasanalyse in der Medizin. *Techn. Messen*, **52**, 247–252 (1985)
18. Gravenstein, J. S. *Gas Monitoring and Pulse Oximetry*, Butterworth-Heinemann, Boston (1990)
19. Bengtson, J. P., Bengtsson, J., Bengtsson, A. and Stenqvist, O. Sampled gas need not be returned during low-flow anesthesia. *J. Clin. Monit.*, **9**, 330–334 (1993)
20. Spieß, W. Narkose im Geschlossenem System mit kontinuierlicher inspiratorischer Sauerstoffmessung. *Anaesthesist*, **26**, 503–513 (1977)
21. Block, F. E. Jr. Monitoring the end-tidal concentration of inhalation agents. In *Update on Modern Inhalation Anaesthetics* (eds G. Torri, and G. Damia), Worldwide Medical Communications, New York (1989), pp. 125–129
22. Davey, A., Moyle, J. T. B. and Ward, C. S. *Ward's Anaesthetic Equipment*, 3rd edn, W. B. Saunders, London (1992)
23. Hayes, J. K., Westenskow, D. R. and Jordan, W. S. Continuous monitoring of inspired and end-tidal anesthetic vapor using a piezoelectric detector. *Anesthesiology*, **57**, A180 (1982)
24. Linstromberg, J. W. and J. J. Muir, J. J. Cross-sensitivity in water vapor in the Enström EMMA. *Anesth. Analg.*, **63**, 75–78 (1987)
25. Whitcher, C. Monitoring of anesthetic halocarbons: self-contained ('stand-alone') equipment. *Sem. Anesth.*, **5**, 213–223 (1986)
26. Cooper, J. B., Newborner, R. S. and Kitz, R. J. An analysis of major errors and equipment failures in anesthesia management: considerations for prevention and detection. *Anesthesiology*, **60**, 34–42 (1984)
27. Lotz, P. Sicherheitstechnische Aspekte bei der Anwendung medizinischtechnischer Geräte im Krankenhaus. *mt-Medizintechnik*, **104**, 133–137 (1984)
28. Baum, J. Kapnometrie und Kapnographie als Sicherheitsfaktoren in der Anästhesie. *Anaesthesiol. Reanimat.*, **16**, 12–22 (1991)
29. Kalenda, Z. *Mastering Infrared Capnography*, Kerkebosch BV, Zeist (1989)
30. Baum, J. and Sachs, G. Frischgasflow und Narkosebeatmung – Technische Voraussetzungen für die adäquate Nutzung von Rückatemsystemen. *Anästh. Intensivther. Notfallmed*, **25**, 72–78 (1990)
31. Lenz, G., Klöss Th. and Schorer, R. Grundlagen und Anwendung der Kapnometrie. *Anästh. Intensivmed.*, **26**, 133–141 (1985)
32. Lindahl, S. G. E., Yates, A. P. and Hatch, D. J. Relationship between invasive and noninvasive measurements of gas exchange in anesthetized infants and children. *Anesthesiology*, **66**, 168–175 (1987)
33. Badgwell, J. M., Heavner, J. E., May, W. S., Goldthorn, J. F. and Lerman, J. End-tidal PCO$_2$ monitoring in infants and children ventilated with either a partial rebreathing or a non-rebreathing circuit. *Anesthesiology*, **66**, 405–410 (1987)
34. Lenz, G., Heipertz, W., Leidig, E. and Madee, S. Intraoperatives Monitoring der Beatmung bei Früh- und Neugeborenen. *Anästh. Intensivther. Notfallmed.*, **21**, 122–126 (1986)
35. Spoerel, W. E. Ist Atemkalk überflüssig? *Anaesthesist*, **26**, 518–524 (1977)
36. Baum, J., Enzenauer, J., Krausse, Th. and Sachs, G. Atemkalk – Nutzungsdauer, Kosten und Verbrauch in Abhängigkeit vom Frischgasfluß. *Anaesthesiol. Reanimat*, **18**, 108–113 (1993)
37. Tinker, J. H., Dull, D. L., Caplan, R. A., Ward, R. J. and Cheney, F. W. Role of monitoring devices in prevention of anesthetic mishaps: a closed claims analysis. *Anesthesiology*, **71**, 541–546 (1989)
38. Gravenstein, J. S. and Paulus, D. A. *Praxis der Patientenüberwachung*, Gustav Fischer Verlag, Stuttgart (1985)

39. Sodal, I. E. and Swanson, G. D. Mass spectrometry: current technology and implications for anesthesia. In *Low Flow and Closed System Anesthesia* (eds J. A. Aldrete, H. J. Lowe and R. W. Virtue), Grune and Stratton, New York (1979), pp. 167–182

40. Weingarten, M. Synopsis of the application of the mass spectrometer to the practice of anesthesia. In *Low Flow and Closed System Anesthesia* (eds J. A. Aldrete, H. J. Lowe and R. W. Virtue), Grune and Stratton, New York (1979), pp. 183–191

41. Walder, B., Lauber, R. and Zbinden, A. M. Genauigkeit und Kreuzempfindlichkeit von volatilen Anästhetika-Analysatoren. *Anaesthesist*, **40** (Suppl. 2), S151 (1991)

9

Patient safety aspects of low flow anaesthesia

In this chapter the prejudices against low flow anaesthesia will be discussed comprehensively. They are the main opposition to a judicious use of technically advanced rebreathing systems by adequate flow reduction. To illustrate the problem, reference will primarily be made to minimal flow anaesthesia, which is a low flow technique practicable in clinical routine, although the flow is virtually reduced to the minimum possible.

9.1 Specific risks of anaesthetic techniques with reduced fresh gas flow

9.1.1 Risks attributable to inadequate technical equipment

The requirements concerning technical equipment have already been subject to extensive discussion (see Chapters 7 and 8). Once more it should be pointed out that the extent of safety facilities for anaesthetic machines is specified by different national standards and in future will be subject to a common European norm. Thus, only those potential risks directly resulting from the reduction of fresh gas flow and the corresponding increase of the rebreathing volume will be discussed.

9.1.1.1 Hypoxia

It cannot be denied that the preconditions for performance of low flow anaesthesia are not ideal if the flow control systems of older anaesthesia machines do not meet the specifications quoted by the manufacturer in the low flow range (see Section 7.2.2). For anaesthesia management with reduced fresh gas flow, the German Dräger company offers optionally to replace old unsuitable flowmeters by special low flow tubes (see Figure 7.1). Furthermore, non-precise adjustment of the flow controls, due to bad performance of the fine needle valves, is liable to cause unexpected alterations of the inspired oxygen concentration and hence possibly hypoxia. In older anaesthetic machines, insufficient gas tightness with corresponding higher loss of gas via leaks, as well as poor fresh gas utilization of older type breathing systems, may be the cause of unexpected decrease of the inspired oxygen concentration. However, under the provisions of many national safety standards, continuous monitoring of the oxygen concentration is mandatory during performance of inhalational anaesthesia. With correct setting of the lower alarm limit, there is no procedure-specific risk involved for the patient. If required, the fresh gas flow and its composition have to be adapted to the specific properties of the available equipment.

9.1.1.2   *Hypoventilation and alterations in ventilation patterns*

Volume shortage in the breathing system resulting from excessive leakage losses will cause a reduction of the ventilatory minute volume and possibly even a change in the ventilation pattern. This is the reason why all anaesthetic machines, breathing systems and ventilators should be subjected to a leak test before minimal flow anaesthesia is implemented. It should be guaranteed at the least that the leakage tolerances quoted by the manufacturer are not exceeded. In the common European standard, maximum tolerances of leakage gas loss at a defined pressure will be established.

An essential shortcoming of conventional anaesthetic machines is the aforementioned linkage between tidal and fresh gas volume (see Section 7.2.6). As the fresh gas flow is reduced so the tidal volume is likewise diminished, since the gas volume which is fed into the system during inspiration decreases. In clinical routine, reduction of the fresh gas flow from 4.4 to 0.5 l/min decreases the minute volume of a normal-weight adult patient by an average of 0.6–1.2 litres. From a clinical point of view, this merely results in a normalization of ventilation for most of the patients, as common routine preadjustment of ventilation causes a more or less significant hyperventilation. Otherwise, the reduction of the ventilation volume can be recognized immediately by means of the mandatory continuous monitoring of the expired volume, and corrected by increasing the tidal volume.

If using low fresh gas volumes, additional gas loss via leakages results in a further decrease of gas volume circulating in the system, thus prompting hypoventilation and possibly alternating pressure ventilation. This in turn can be detected sufficiently early by the mandatory airway pressure monitoring. Provided that the disconnection alarm is adjusted correctly to slightly below the peak pressure, hypoventilation resulting from gas volume deficiency will cause an immediate alarm.

Basically, high leakage gas losses involve the risk of alterations in the ventilatory patterns in addition to the corresponding hypoventilation. However, this can be rapidly recognized and corrected when monitoring standards are followed. Anaesthetic machines with an anaesthetic gas reservoir are far better suited for use with low fresh gas flows, and the problems described will not arise as long as the reservoir is filled sufficiently. Essentially, all problems resulting from leakage gas loss can be minimized by appropriate maintenance of the anaesthetic machines.

9.1.1.3   *Carbon dioxide accumulation in the breathing system*

In contrast to high flow anaesthesia, efficient carbon dioxide elimination is an essential in the performance of anaesthesia with low fresh gas flow since, with the increase in rebreathing volume, the carbon dioxide concentration in the breathing system may rise considerably if the absorbers are exhausted (see Figure 8.8).

According to the author's own investigations, the usage period of absorbers filled with pelleted soda lime is considerably longer than previously quoted in relevant textbooks (see Section 7.2.5.1). If suitable carbon dioxide monitoring is available (see Section 8.6.2), the soda lime should not be discarded routinely, but preferably be used until it is completely exhausted. But if an anaesthetic machine is used which does not permit constant carbon dioxide measurement, use should be made of double canisters or Jumbo absorbers and the soda lime should be discarded routinely, at least whenever a colour change of the indicator signals the beginning of exhaustion. Proceeding in this way, the patient is reliably protected from carbon dioxide rebreathing[1].

9.1.1.4 Accidental increase of the airway pressure

In some anaesthetic ventilators, such as the Megamed 700 (Megamed, Cham, Switzerland), the excess gas is not discharged via an automatically opening spill valve but via an overflow valve, which is operated manually. Working with extremely low flows, this valve needs to be closed virtually completely. If this valve is not appropriately adjusted to the fresh gas flow and the loss of gas volume resulting from uptake and leaks, this may cause either gas volume shortage or the development of an increasing positive pressure within the breathing system. This fault in operating the machine will also soon be detected if occlusion and disconnection alarms are set appropriately. Another safety feature to prevent an accidental barotrauma is the airway pressure limit valve (APL valve) which opens automatically if a preadjusted positive pressure within the breathing system is reached.

9.1.1.5 Accidental overdose of volatile anaesthetics

Even in severe misadjustment of plenum vaporizers outside the circle, it is virtually impossible that this will result in a rapidly occurring overdose during low flow anaesthesia. On the one hand, this can be attributed to the link between the vaporizer output and the fresh gas flow; on the other hand, to the fact that, due to different safety regulations, the output of nearly all vaporizers is limited. In low flow anaesthesia, alterations of the anaesthetic concentration proceed very slowly due to the long time constant of the breathing system (Figure 9.1a,b). In the event of accidental maladjustment, changes in volatile agent concentration can always be recognized sufficiently early by means of careful clinical observation of the patient. Increase in rebreathing volume does not involve a higher risk of overdose of inhalational anaesthetic.

From this point of view, this procedure is evidently safer than anaesthesia with high fresh gas flow where accidental adjustment errors at the vaporizer result in immediate drastic changes of the anaesthetic concentration in the breathing system.

It has been pointed out before (see Section 8.4) that a change from low to high fresh gas flow may result in serious overdose if the setting at the vaporizer is not readjusted appropriately to the higher flow with its shorter time

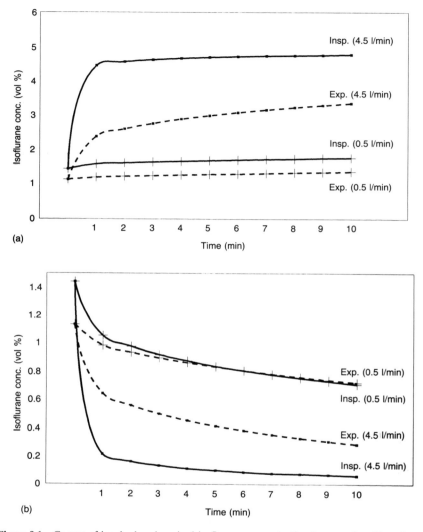

Figure 9.1 Course of inspired and expired isoflurane concentration in case of accidental adjustment error of the vaporizer: (a) vaporizer accidentally set to its maximum output; (b) vaporizer accidentally closed (Patient 75 kg, AMV 5.6 l/min (GUS))

constant. This is the reason why anaesthesia using a flow lower than 1 l/min should not be performed without continuously monitoring the anaesthetic concentration in the breathing system. Once more it should be pointed out that continuous monitoring of inhalation anaesthetic concentration will be obligatory under the forthcoming European standard demanding all inhalation anaesthetic machines to be equipped with this safety facility.

9.1.2   Risks which are directly caused by reduction of the fresh gas flow

9.1.2.1   The long time constant

The assumption that the long time constant poses a specific risk due to the inability to rapidly change the anaesthetic gas composition if required during low flow anaesthesia is absolutely unfounded. A desired gas composition can be immediately attained at any time by switching to a high fresh gas flow to shorten the time constant of the breathing system. This approach is especially recommended to those anaesthetists who are on the verge of gaining initial experience with minimal flow anaesthesia. Once familiar with the technique, rapid increase of anaesthetic depth can be achieved by intravenous injection of supplementary drugs. Rapid lightening of the anaesthetic, on the other hand, can only be achieved by increasing the fresh gas flow.

It will only be possible to rapidly reduce the concentration of volatile anaesthetic while maintaining low flow if the anaesthetic machine is equipped with a charcoal absorber (see Section 7.3.1). The anaesthetic concentration will drop instantly whenever the absorber is switched into the breathing system (Figure 9.2)[2,3].

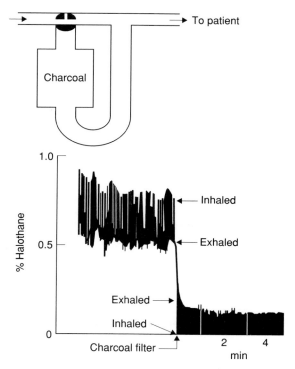

Figure 9.2   Charcoal filter, switched by bypass into the breathing system, for rapid elimination of inhalational anaesthetics in low flow anaesthetic techniques (From Ernst and Spain[55], by permission)

9.1.2.2   Accumulation of foreign gas

9.1.2.2.1   NITROGEN

For a patient of normal weight, the nitrogen volume stored in the body and in the lungs can be assumed as being 2.7 litres. If denitrogenation is performed over a period of 15–20 min with high fresh gas flow, a volume of about 2 litres nitrogen is washed out of all compartments during this period. The remaining 0.7 litre is only slowly released from the less perfused tissues[4,5]. If the fresh gas flow is reduced to extremely low values after such an apparently sufficient denitrogenation, the nitrogen concentration in the breathing system will rise to about 3–10% within the next hour[4,6–12]. Nitrogen accumulation in the breathing system may increase even more if side-stream gas analysers are used, since considerable volumes of ambient air, which serves as calibration or reference gas, may be returned into the system together with the sampling gas. Depending on the volume of ambient air admixed to the sampling gas and the degree of flow reduction, nitrogen concentrations of 15% or even higher can be observed in the case of long-term minimal flow anaesthesia (see Sections 7.3.1, 8.2.1, 8.5 and 8.7). Should undesirable nitrogen concentrations be reached in the breathing system, nitrogen can be washed out by a 2–5 min flushing phase with high fresh gas flow[7–9,13]. During anaesthesia, accumulation of nitrogen in the system can only be detected by means of a mass spectrometer or a multi-gas analyser. It must be emphasized, however, that nitrogen accumulation does not involve any risk for the patient as long as hypoxia can be definitely excluded, though the nitrous oxide concentration may be reduced considerably, thus lessening its analgesic effects[7]. To ensure sufficient analysis nitrous oxide concentration from time to time appropriate correction of the anaesthetic gas composition by intermittent flushing with high fresh gas flow may be carried out, or anaesthesia has to be completed by supplementary administration of intravenous or volatile anaesthetics.

9.1.2.2.2   ACETONE

Acetone is generated by the oxidative metabolism of free fatty acids. Increased formation may be observed in the state of starvation, in decompensated diabetes mellitus, and in the case of an increased release of anti-insulin hormones. If isoflurane anaesthesia with closed system is performed over a period of 6 h, an average increase of acetone blood concentration of 50 mg/l and, in individual cases, of up to 200 mg/l was observed[14]. The increase in acetone concentration during closed system anaesthesia depends on its preoperative value and on the duration of the anaesthetic procedure[15,16]. A blood concentration higher than 50 mg/l[15] is said to extend the emergence period and to be liable to increase postoperative vomiting. In performing anaesthesia with closed system over a period of 4 h, Morita et al.[9] revealed an average increase of acetone concentration from 1.3 to 5.9 ppm in the breathing gas. The MAK value (German list of maximum workplace concentrations) assessed for acetone is 1000 ppm, the normal value for blood concentration less than 5 mg/l, the limit value tolerated with respect to industrial hygiene is 20 mg/l. However, the US Navy concentration limit for acetone in ambient air in submarines is established at even 2000 ppm over a period of 24 h[17].

Furthermore, it has to be emphasized that even with the use of semi-open breathing systems considerable increase of blood acetone concentration cannot be prevented. During the first 5 h of anaesthesia, Strauß et al.[16] could not establish a significant difference when comparing the use of closed and semi-open breathing systems. Differences only became clinically relevant after 6 h anaesthesia (Figure 9.3).

Because of its particular solubility in water and fat, the acetone concentration cannot be lowered by means of intermittent short-term high flow flushing phases[9]. For safety reasons the author recommends, in patients suffering from decompensated diabetes mellitus and patients with otherwise raised blood acetone concentration, not to use fresh gas flows lower than 1 l/min during long-term anaesthesia. By the resulting continuous flush effect, undesired trace gas accumulation can be prevented. Intraoperative stress which promotes endogenous acetone production can be decreased in long-term anaesthesia by additional application of opioids, in accordance with the concept of balanced anaesthesia.

9.1.2.2.3   ETHANOL

Ethanol, with a gas–water solubility coefficient of 1200, may accumulate in the closed system similarly to acetone, and its concentration in the breathing gas can barely be decreased by short-term intermittent flushing phases[9]. However, high ethanol concentrations result exclusively from exogenous intoxication. If a surgical intervention has to be performed urgently on an alcoholized patient, elimination of ethanol by exhalation would be made impossible by anaesthesia with a closed system. Again it seems prudent in these cases not to reduce the fresh gas flow to below 1 l/min in order to provide an adequate wash-out effect.

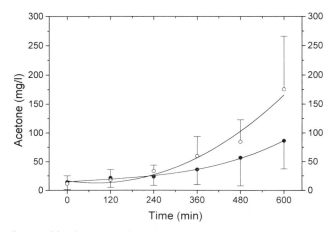

Figure 9.3   Acetone blood concentrations during the course of anaesthesia: ● semi-open breathing system, ○ closed rebreathing system. Regression curves (normal value: 170 mol/l) (From Strauß et al.[18], by permission)

9.1.2.2.4 CARBON MONOXIDE

During performance of anaesthesia with a closed system over a period of 2 h, the carbon monoxide concentration in the breathing system was found to increase to an average of 80 ppm within the range of 20–210 ppm[19]. The values measured for non-smokers after 6 h anaesthesia with closed system amounted to 0.5–1.5% carbon monoxide haemoglobin (COHb), while for smokers the values reached 3% COHb. The average increase for both groups amounted to 0.4% COHb, but in an individual case an increase of up to 3.5% COHb was observed[18].

The physiological value of COHb amounts to 0.4–0.8%, but with habitual smokers this value may reach 10%. Concentrations of 100 ppm over an exposure period of 8 h, and 400 ppm over a period of 1 h, are considered hazardous. The toxicity of carbon monoxide can be estimated with the Henderson and Haggard toxicity index (I_{tox})[19]:

$$I_{tox} = C_{CO} \times t$$

where C_{CO} = carbon monoxide concentration (ppm)
　　　t　　= exposure period (hours).

No effects were observed with an I_{tox} of 300 ppmh, symptoms of beginning intoxication with 600 ppmh, vomiting and headache with 900 ppmh; a value of 1500 ppmh is life-threatening. Middleton *et al.*[19] point out that, in the case of closed system anaesthesia, a toxicity index of about 200–300 ppmh is reached.

Only a very small volume of carbon monoxide (0.42 ± 0.07 ml/h) is endogenously produced under normal conditions. However, in the closed system, the concentration may rise to values of clinical relevance in the case of heavy smokers, haemolysis, anaemia, porphyria and blood transfusions, particularly when blood donated by smokers is given. Where high risk patients are concerned, such as heavy smokers suffering from severe anaemia with considerable regional perfusion restriction, low flow anaesthesia should be performed in preference to closed system anaesthesia to ensure continuous wash-out of carbon monoxide[18,19]. Due to its high affinity for haemoglobin, intermittent short flushing with high fresh gas flow will be insufficient as only the amount of carbon monoxide within the gas-containing space (lung and breathing system) is expelled. As soon as the flow is reduced again, the carbon monoxide concentration will slowly be re-established, balancing the partial pressure difference.

Moon reported several cases of intraoperative carbon monoxide poisoning which were held to be caused by carbon monoxide generation in carbon dioxide absorbent following exposure to fluorinated anaesthetics[20,21]. Canisters which had been in place for longer periods of time were more likely to contain high carbon monoxide concentrations. This phenomenon could be observed with the use of both baralyme and soda lime. To avoid carbon monoxide intoxication, the use of high fresh gas flows and frequent changes of the absorbent were recommended[22]. In a clinical trial of more than 1000 unselected patients[23], in no case could dangerous or excessive carbon monoxide hemoglobin concentrations be found, although minimal flow anaesthesia was performed routinely and the absorbent canisters were used for several days (Figure 9.4). As revealed by Fang and Eger[24], only

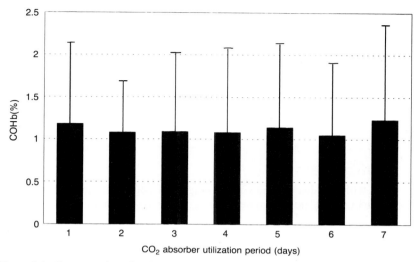

Figure 9.4   Concentration of carbon monoxide haemoglobin as a function of the carbon dioxide absorber's utilization period. All blood samples were taken at least 20 min after fresh gas flow reduction to 0.5 l/min

absolutely dry absorbents produce carbon monoxide when exposed to volatile anaesthetics containing a CHF_2 moiety, like enflurane, isoflurane and desflurane. Barium hydroxide lime is more liable than soda lime to generate carbon monoxide. Thus, all measures that dry out the absorbent must be carefully avoided. Quite contrary to Moon's assumptions, low flow anaesthetic techniques protect from carbon monoxide generation, as they preserve the moisture content of the absorbent. Accordingly, there is no particular risk of accidental occurrence of hazardous carbon monoxide concentrations in low flow anaesthesia[56].

9.1.2.2.5   METHANE

Methane, which is generated in the intestines by bacterial decomposition processes, is a physiological constituent of intestinal gases. It may accumulate in the anaesthetic gas during anaesthesia with closed system[4]. The average methane concentration measured after 2 h anaesthesia amounted to 11.2 ppm. The maximum value measured in an individual case was 229 ppm. Methane concentrations of up to 100 ppm are found in the expired air of healthy test persons. Being a non-toxic trace gas, methane is of significance only in so far as it is flammable if mixed with oxygen (5–60% in oxygen) or nitrous oxide (4–40% in nitrous oxide). But such methane concentrations are not obtained even in long-term closed system anaesthesia[25].

Rolly, however, recently published observations gained during performance of total intravenous anaesthesia on patients being ventilated with an oxygen–air mixture with the aid of the closed circuit PhysioFlex apparatus (Physio, Haarlem, The Netherlands). Although a volatile agent was not used, the inbuilt infrared analyser indicated unexpected values for halothane in patients undergoing gynaecological laparoscopies with carbon dioxide insufflation[26]. The mean concentration of methane was 861 ppm, ranging from 139 to 1967 ppm in closed system anaesthesia lasting from 45 to 150 min. Thus, the methane concentrations were much higher than mentioned previously. Rolly concludes that these high methane concentrations exert considerable influence on the infrared absorption analysis of halothane, with 800 ppm being interpreted as 1% halothane by the measuring device. That calls into question the closed loop feedback control of halothane administration based on infrared absorption measurement.

9.1.2.2.6   HYDROGEN

Hydrogen, which is discharged via the lungs in a volume of up to 0.6 ml/min, also may accumulate in the anaesthetic gas during anaesthesia with closed system. On average, the concentration rises by 200 ppm/h[27]. However, flammable hydrogen concentrations (4.6–94% in oxygen, 5.8–86% in nitrous oxide) are likewise not reached in long-term anaesthesia with closed systems.

9.1.2.2.7   DEGRADATION PRODUCTS OF VOLATILE ANAESTHETICS RESULTING FROM CHEMICAL REACTION WITH CARBON DIOXIDE ABSORBENTS

2-Bromo-2-chloro-1,1-difluoroethylene, CF_2CBrCl, a gaseous decomposition product of halothane, may reach concentrations of 4–5 ppm with a closed system[28]. Experiments with model rebreathing systems indicate that 0.02% of the halothane is transformed into CF_2CBrCl within 4 h. Although the levels of CF_2CBrCl, gained during 1 h of closed system anaesthesia are significantly less than the toxic concentration, quoted as 250 ppm according to Sharp, these findings do raise concern regarding the use of closed circuit halothane administration.

Sevoflurane reacts with carbon dioxide absorbents by formation of fluoromethyl-2,2-difluoro-1-(trifluoromethyl) vinyl ether (compound A) and fluoromethyl-2-methoxy-2,2-difluoro-1-(trifluoromethyl) ethyl ether (compound B); the degradation is considerably promoted by the heat which develops in the carbon dioxide absorber[29]. If anaesthesia was performed with a semi-closed system, concentrations of compound A in the breathing gas amounted to about 4 ppm. On the contrary, in anaesthesia with low fresh gas flow of about 0.8 l/min, mean maximum inspired concentration of compound A using barium hydroxide lime was 20.3 ± 8.6 ppm compared to 8.16 ± 2.67 ppm obtained with soda lime after 4 h. In an individual case, a maximum concentration of 60.78 ppm was reached during low flow anaesthesia with barium hydroxide lime[30]. These concentrations are considered to be of no clinical relevance, as sevoflurane, if used in low flow circuit for 3–5 h duration, generally produces only low levels of degradation compound A, being well below the concentration reported to cause toxicity (LC_{50} in rats, 400–420 ppm after 3 h exposure[29]), But the authors admit that further studies will be needed to evaluate potential variability in compound A production. In an abstract published recently, higher concentrations of sevoflurane degradation products were found in animal experiments. During

6 h closed system anaesthesia with barium hydroxide lime and 1.5 MAC sevoflurane, compound A reached a concentration of 90 ± 19 ppm and compound B 35 ± 15 ppm[31]. Japanese authors established concentrations between 10 and 25 ppm in the anaesthetic gas after 60 min of low flow anaesthesia, and 37.5 ppm after 150 min. They also assume these concentration to be of no clinical relevance and consider low flow anaesthesia with sevoflurane up to a duration of 2 h to be justifiable, especially as the high humidity, which is typical of low flow anaesthesia, reduces degradation of sevoflurane[32]. The American Food and Drug Administration (FDA) demands a fresh gas flow rate of at least 2 l/min if sevoflurane is administered via a rebreathing system.

9.1.2.2.8   IMPLICATIONS FOR ANAESTHETIC PRACTICE

Foreign gases may accumulate in the breathing system if anaesthesia is performed with extremely low fresh gas flows. These are gases which

- are formed in the body, such as acetone, carbon monoxide, methane, hydrogen and gaseous metabolites of inhalation agents
- are absorbed by the body, stored in the tissues and discharged via the lungs, such as ethanol, carbon monoxide and nitrogen
- are either generated in the system, or fed into the breathing system as contaminants together with the fresh or the sampling gas, such as carbon monoxide, degradation products of sevoflurane and halothane with carbon dioxide absorbents, nitrogen and argon[9,57] (Table 9.1).

Sparingly soluble gases, such as nitrogen, methane and hydrogen, can be washed out from the system, if required, by brief intermittent flushing with a high fresh gas flow. But if gases readily soluble in water and fat, such as acetone and alcohol, accumulate within the breathing system, anaesthesia on high risk patients should preferably be performed with semi-closed rebreathing systems and continuous discharge of excess gas, at least with

Table 9.1   Contaminants of medical gases*

	Oxygen for medical use	Nitrous oxide for anaesthesia
$Ar + N_2$	≈ 5000 ppm	
CO	< 5 ppm	< 10 ppm
CO_2	< 50 ppm	< 300 ppm
Halogens		< 5 ppm
H_2S		< 1 ppm
NH_3	< 1 ppm	< 5 ppm
NO/NO_2	< 1 ppm	< 5 ppm
Cl_2	< 0.5 ppm	
SO_2	< 1 ppm	
$N_2 + O_2$		≈ 4600 ppm

*The low concentrations of O_2 contaminants meet the requirements of the German and European Pharmacopoeias, the levels of N_2O contaminants the requirements of the European, US and German Pharmacopoeias (Source: Messer Griesheim, Frankfurt a. Main, Germany).

low flow anaesthesia. This ensures that these foreign gases are continuously washed out from the breathing system.

The same recommendation applies for gases characterized by high affinity for the tissues or blood, like carbon monoxide. High risk patients, such as heavy smokers suffering from severe regionally restricted perfusion undergoing mass transfusions, preferably should be anaesthetized using semi-closed rebreathing systems with a fresh gas flow of at least 1 l/min, thus realizing a sufficient wash-out effect.

Concerning inhalation anaesthetics such as halothane and sevoflurane, which are subject to degradation by carbon dioxide absorbents, these agents should not for safety reasons[28,33] be administered using closed or minimal flow anaesthesia, but preferably should be given via semi-closed rebreathing systems with a fresh gas flow of at least 1–2 l/min.

Nevertheless, although foreign gas accumulation needs to be considered thoroughly, the author agrees with Baumgarten and Reynolds[17] that the trace gas issue cannot '... justify the continued waste and pollution of high flow anaesthesia'.

9.2   Specific safety features of anaesthetic techniques with reduced fresh gas flow

9.2.1   Improved equipment maintenance

The increased demands placed on the technical equipment call for more painstaking care, maintenance and testing of anaesthetic machines. When technical inspections are carried out, particular interest should be focused upon testing the equipment in the lower flow ranges to ensure that it at least meets the technical specifications of the manufacturer. The equipment should be carefully tested and readjusted if required over the entire specified operation range as given in the service manuals. There cannot be any doubt that the high demands placed on equipment care and maintenance are an essential factor in terms of patient safety. It must be emphasized that it is the anaesthetist who is ultimately responsible for careful handling and maintenance of anaesthetic equipment[34], to avoid technical complications like those described in detail by Müchler[35], Good[36] and Johnstone[37].

9.2.2   The long time constant

The long time constant of the breathing system[38] is an extraordinary safety factor in low flow anaesthesia. Schreiber[39,40] analyses a potentially hazardous situation threatening the patient's safety as consisting of different periods (Figure 9.5):

● pre-alarm period: the time from occurrence of an adverse condition to the generation of the alarm (A–B)
● Identification period: the time it takes on the part of the anaesthetist to identify the origin of the alarm (B–C); it takes some further time for the anaesthetist to identify exactly the cause of the alarm (C–D)

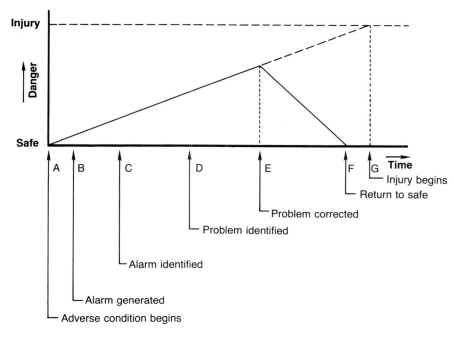

Figure 9.5 Analysis of a critical incident: A–B, pre-alarm period; B–D, identification period; D–E, correction period; E–F, restitution period; B–G, reaction period – the time from onset of the alarm to definite injury (From Schreiber and Schreiber[40], by permission)

- Correction period: after having analysed the particular cause of the problem, it takes some time for the corrective action to be carried out and the system starts with its corresponding reaction (D–E)
- Restitution period: the time which elapses until the system returns to its safe starting condition (E–F).

If any of these phases of a critical incident is prolonged, the danger to the patient may escalate to that point where injury cannot be prevented by correcting measures (G). The time from the generation of an alarm to the actual occurrence of an injury is referred to as the reaction period (B–G). This is the period that the anaesthetist has available as a maximum to protect the patient from being injured.

The increase in safety achieved by the long time constants, especially in minimal flow anaesthesia can be impressively demonstrated by a clinical example. The following situation was simulated on a young healthy male patient in the presence of two anaesthetists (Figure 9.6).

During anaesthesia, and starting each time with an inspired oxygen concentration of 32% at steady-state conditions, the oxygen supply was interrupted while the nitrous oxide supply remained unchanged. This test was performed with different fresh gas flows of 6, 3, 1 and 0.5 l/min. The lower alarm limit of the oxygen monitor was set to 28%. The test was interrupted immediately if an inspired oxygen concentration of 22% was

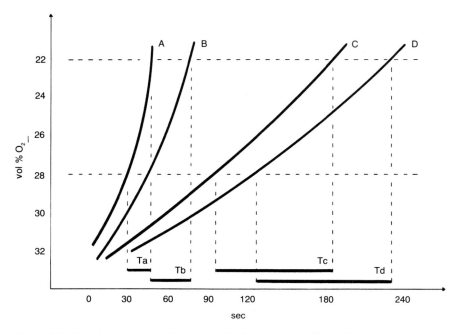

Figure 9.6 Reaction period as a function of the fresh gas flow. Simulation of accidental interruption of oxygen flow on an anaesthetic machine without oxygen ratio controller. With low fresh gas flows (Tc and Td), the reaction period takes considerably longer than with high fresh gas flows (Ta and Tb). Fresh gas flow: A = 6 l/min, B = 3 l/min, C = 1 l/min, D = 0.5 l/min

reached, and the breathing system flushed with pure oxygen. In this test, the oxygen concentration of 22% will represent the critical limit at which potential injury may endanger the patient.

It can clearly be recognized from the illustration that, with a fresh gas flow of 1.0 or 0.5 l/min, the reaction period (Tc and Td) is considerably longer than with a high fresh gas flow of 6 or 3 l/min (Ta and Tb). This in turn means that with low fresh gas flow considerably more time is left for identification and correction of an operating error than with high fresh gas flow. The long time constants of low flow anaesthesia are a specific safety factor which is directly based on the reduction of the fresh gas flow. It prevents sudden accidental hypoxia or anaesthetic agent misdosage in case of inadvertent errors in operating the anaesthetic machine. As regards this point, low flow anaesthetic techniques definitely involve less risks than anaesthesia with high fresh gas flow.

9.2.3   Improved knowledge of the theory and practice of inhalation anaesthesia

An essential safety factor will be improved knowledge about inhalation anaesthesia gained by dealing with the theoretical basis and clinical characteristics of low flow anaesthetic techniques. Prior to performance of such methods, the anaesthetist has to be committed to many specific aspects of anaesthesia. This in turn enhances the understanding of kinetic uptake processes during the course of anaesthesia and of the technical details and features of the anaesthetic machines.

It is self-evident that the early period of training, when first experiences are gained with this technique, requires increased attention to the observation of both patient and machine. But in no way can it be claimed that such increased care and attention during anaesthesia should be considered a disadvantage of the method[41]. On the contrary, increased care and attention reduces the risk involved for the patient. Whenever the anaesthetist feels overstrained in a certain clinical situation, he or she is free at any time to switch back to high fresh gas flow and to continue anaesthesia using a more familiar method.

It can be emphasized from the author's own experience that, in dealing with low flow techniques, the anaesthetist learns much about both the patients and the anaesthetic machine[42,43]. This corresponds with the observation published by Deshane and Edsall[44]. The incidence of hypoxaemia with the use of nitrous oxide and varying fresh gas flows during general anaesthetic maintenance were retrospectively studied using computerized patient records on 1064 patients. No hypoxaemia occurred with fresh gas flow less than $3 \, l/min$ and the incidence of expired oxygen concentration lower than 26% was significantly ($p < 0.20$) greater with fresh gas flow higher than $3 \, l/min$. The reported results support the thesis that performance of low flow techniques results in increased appreciation of problems and correspondingly careful management of anaesthesia.

9.3   Implications for anaesthetic practice

The potential risks involved in reduction of the fresh gas flow nowadays can always be detected early due to the safety features (Table 9.2) specified by different technical standards and regulations. The performance of low flow anaesthetic techniques thus does not specifically increase the risk for the

Table 9.2   Safety features of inhalation anaesthetic machines (as required by the forthcoming common European standard)

Oxygen supply pressure alarm
Nitrous oxide cut-off
Oxygen bypass
Oxygen ratio controller
Device for single vaporizer operation
Monitoring of inspired oxygen concentration
Airway pressure monitoring
Disconnection alarm
Occlusion alarm
Monitoring of exhaled volume
Alternative monitoring of ventilation: carbon dioxide monitoring
Monitoring of volatile anaesthetic concentration

patient, and, if anaesthetic machines of the new generation are available, generally will not require additional monitoring.

It must be pointed out, however, that conventional anaesthesia machines with continuous fresh gas supply, featuring an anaesthetic ventilator with hanging bellows, are inadequate in terms both of guaranteeing a constant gas volume during mechanical ventilation and with respect to the precision of the flow control systems. Only machines of the new generation satisfy completely all the technical requirements which facilitate anaesthesia with maximally reduced fresh gas flows. Essential technical features are the discontinuous supply of fresh gas into the breathing system and the existence of an anaesthetic gas reservoir. By these technical details the minor volume imbalances which typically occur with minimal flow anaesthesia are compensated for. Anaesthetic machines, specifically designed for the use of low fresh gas flows and for judicious use of rebreathing technique, do not present any problems in the routine performance even of minimal flow anaesthesia. If, however, use is made of the older conventional machines mentioned above, performance of this anaesthetic method calls for careful observation of ventilation parameters and may need more readjustments in machine settings.

Essentially, the risk involved for the patient during anaesthesia depends on the anaesthetist's familiarity with the anaesthetic method selected and his knowledge regarding the procedure-specific potential complications[45].

It has been proved that only about 4–11% of anaesthetic incidents are definitely caused by malfunction of equipment[34,40,46,47], while 70–80% must be attributed to human error[40,48–50]. Complications are frequently correlated

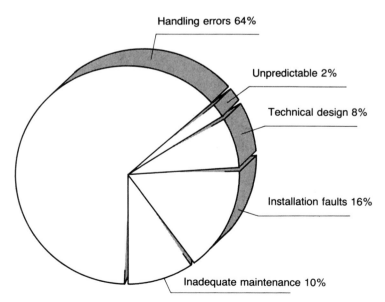

Figure 9.7   Causes of incidents with technical equipment used in medicine (From Lotz[46], by permission)

with inadequate equipment testing and maintenance, insufficient knowledge and familiarity with the machine and the anaesthetic method plus wrong operation of the controls (Figure 9.7). Calkins[48] points out that complications may arise, in particular, if the interactions between breathing system and anaesthesia machine are misjudged.

The following conclusions may be drawn from these points of discussion:

1. Dealing with low flow anaesthetic methods should be made a rule in the training of young anaesthetists. Improved understanding of technical and physiological processes during inhalation anaesthesia provides an essential safety factor for the patient.
2. Young anaesthetists who are still in the training phase should perform low flow techniques only under the supervision of an experienced consultant. This is even more important if the mechanical equipment does not perfectly satisfy all the ideal technical requirements of this method.
3. In the management of critical situations and patients, the anaesthetists should adhere to that method in which they are best trained and familiarized. To proceed in this manner always reduces the risk to the patient.
4. Selection of the fresh gas flow should be flexibly adapted to the respective conditions which are a function of the surgical procedure, the equipment and the anaesthetist's state of training.
5. The safety of the patient must always assume first priority in the anaesthetist's decision concerning the anaesthetic method[41,51].

If these self-evident rules are borne in mind when a decision is made in favour of an anaesthetic method, low flow anaesthesia can be understood as an alternative technique just as safe as anaesthesia with high fresh gas flow[42,52-54]. But it is only with minimal and low flow anaesthesia that the advantages of rebreathing rendered by the sophisticated technical standards of present-day anaesthetic machines can be used to their best potential.

9.4   Contraindications for low flow anaesthetic techniques

9.4.1   Relative contraindications

In inhalation anaesthesia lasting less than 15 min, fresh gas flow reduction is unsuitable, because there is an increased risk of:

- insufficient denitrogenation
- insufficiently rapid initial increase of anaesthetic depth
- gas volume deficiency.

If the breathing system cannot be kept sufficiently gas tight, fresh gas flow reduction may be impossible:

- in case of rigid bronchoscopy
- when using uncuffed endotracheal tubes
- when using non-rebreathing systems, for instance during magnetic resonance imaging
- when using insufficiently gas-tight breathing systems
- during anaesthesia with a face mask.

If the equipment does not meet essential requirements to ensure patient safety, the fresh gas flow must not be reduced to low values under any circumstances:

● in case of soda lime exhaustion
● in case of failure of the oxygen monitor
● in case of imprecise performance of the gas flow controls.

If there is a risk of accumulation of potentially dangerous trace gases, the fresh gas flow should be at least 1 l/min so as to guarantee a continuous wash-out effect. Such contraindications for the use of extremely low fresh gas flow rates include:

● decompensated diabetes mellitus
● the state of long-term starvation
● anaesthesia performed on chronic alcoholics
● anaesthesia performed on patients with alcohol intoxication
● heavy smokers suffering from severe restriction of regional perfusion
● the use of halothane – if sevoflurane is used, the American Food and Drug Administration even suggests a flow of at least 2 l/min.

9.4.2   Absolute contraindications

The following are absolute contraindications for low flow anaesthetic techniques:

● smoke or gas intoxication
● malignant hyperthermia
● septicaemia
● acute bronchospasm if anaesthetic machines are used which feature anaesthetic ventilators with forced expiratory filling of hanging bellows.

9.5   References

1. Baum, J., Enzenauer, J., Krausse, Th. and Sachs, G. Atemkalk, Nutzungsdauer, Verbrauch und Kosten in Abhängigkeit vom Frischgasfluß. *Anaesthesiol. Reanimat.*, **18**, 108–113 (1993)
2. Ernst, E. A. Use of charcoal to rapidly decrease depth of anesthesia while maintaining a close circuit. *Anesthesiology*, **57**, 343 (1982)
3. Romano, E., Pegoraro, M., Vacri, A., Pecchiari, C. and Auci, E. Low-flow anaesthesia systems, charcoal and isoflurane kinetics. *Anaesthesia*, **47**, 1098–1099 (1992)
4. Barton, F. and Nunn, J. F. Totally closed circuit nitrous oxide/oxygen anaesthesia. *Br. J. Anaesth.*, **47**, 350–357 (1975)
5. Nunn, J. F. Techniques for induction of closed circuit anaesthesia. In *Low Flow and Closed System Anesthesia* (eds J. A. Aldrete, H. J. Lowe and R. W. Virtue) Grune and Stratton, New York (1979), pp. 3–10
6. Barton, F. and Nunn, J. F. Use of refractometry to determine nitrogen accumulation in closed circuits. *Br. J. Anaesth.*, **47**, 346–348 (1975)
7. Bengtson, J. P., Bengtsson, J., Bengtsson, A. and Stenqvist, O. Sampled gas need not be returned during low-flow anesthesia. *J. Clin. Monit.*, **9**, 330–334 (1993)
8. Lin, C. Y., Mostert, J. W. and Benson, D. W. Closed circle systems. A new direction in the practice of anaesthesia. *Acta Anaesth. Scand.*, **24**, 354–361 (1980)

9. Morita, S., Latta, W., Hambro, K. and Snider, M. T. Accumulation of methane, acetone, and nitrogen in the inspired gas during closed-circuit anesthesia. *Anesth. Analg.*, **64**, 343–347 (1985)

10. Versichelen, L. and Rolly, G. Nitrogen accumulation during closed circuit anaesthesia. *Circular*, **6**, 10 (1989)

11. Versichelen, L. and Rolly, G. Mass-spectrometric evaluation of some recently introduced low flow, closed circuit systems. *Acta Anaesth. Belg.*, **41**, 225–237 (1990)

12. Westenskow, D. R., Jordan, W. S. and Gehmlich, D. S. Electronic feedback control and measurement of oxygen consumption during closed circuit anesthesia. In *Low Flow and Closed System Anesthesia* (eds J. A. Aldrete, H. J. Low and R. W. Virtue), Grune and Stratton, New York (1979), pp. 135–146

13. Spieß, W. Narkose im geschlossenen System mit kontinuierlicher inspiratorischer Sauerstoffmessung. *Anaesthesist*, **26**, 503–513 (1977)

14. Strauß, J., Hausdörfer, J., Bannasch, W. and Bang, S. Akkumulation von Aceton während Langzeitnarkosen in halboffenen und geschlossenen Kreissystemen. *Anaesthesist*, **40** (Suppl. 2), S260 (1991)

15. Strauß, J. M. and Hausdörfer, J. Accumulation of acetone in blood during long-term anaesthesia with closed system. *Br. J. Anaesth.*, **70**, 363–364 (1993)

16. Strauß, J. M., Krohn, S. and Sümpelmann, R. Pulmonale Elimination von Azeton und Beatmung im geschlossenen System. *Anaesthesist*, **42** (Suppl. 1), S290 (1993)

17. Baumgarten, R. K. and Reynolds, W. J. Much ado about nothing: trace gaseous metabolites in the closed circuit. *Anesth. Analg.*, **64** 1029–1030 (1985)

18. Strauß, J. M., Bannasch, W., Hausdörfer, J. and Bang, S. Die Entwicklung von Carboxyhämoglobin während Langzeitnarkosen im geschlossenen Kreissystem. *Anaesthesist*, **40**, 324–327 (1991)

19. Middleton, V., van Poznak, A., Artusio, J. R. and Smith, S. M. Carbon monoxide accumulation in closed circle anesthesia systems. *Anesthesiology*, **26**, 715–719 (1965)

20. Moon, R. E., Meyer, A. F., Scott, D. L., Fox, E., Millington, D. S. and Norwood, D. M. Intraoperative carbon monoxide toxicity. *Anesthesiology*, **73** (Suppl. 3A), A1049 (1990)

21. Moon, R. E., Ingram, C., Brunner, E. A. and Meyer, A. F. Spontaneous generation of carbon monoxide within anaesthetic circuits. *Anesthesiology*, **75** (Suppl. ASA Abstracts), A873 (1991)

22. Moon, R. E. Carbon monoxide gas may be linked to CO_2 absorbant. *Anesth. Patient Safety Found. Newslett.*, **6**, 8 (1991)

23. Baum, J., Sachs, G., v.d. Driesch, Ch. and Stanke, H.-G. Carbon monoxide generation in carbon dioxide absorbents. *Anesth. Analg.*, **81**, 144–146 (1995)

24. Fang, Z. X. and Eger II, E. I., Laster, M. J., Chartkoff, B. S., Kandel, L. and Ionescu, P. Carbon monoxide production from degradation of desflurane, enflurane, isoflurane, halothane and sevoflurane by soda lime and baralyme®. *Anesth. Analog.*, **80**, 1187–1193 (1995)

25. Morita, S. Inspired gas contamination by non-anesthetic gases during closed circuit anesthesia. *Circular*, **2**, 24–25 (1985)

26. Rolly, G. and Versichelen, L. Methane accumulation during closed circuit anesthesia. *Anesth. Analg.*, **74** (Suppl.), S253 (1992)

27. Morita, S., Toyooka, H. and Nagase, M. Hydrogen accumulation in closed circuit. *Jap. J. Anesth.*, **34**, 468–472 (1985)

28. Sharp, H. J., Trudell, J. R. and Cohen, E. N. Volatile metabolites and decomposition products of Halothane in man. *Anesthesiology*, **50**, 2–8 (1979)

29. Morio, M., Fujii, K., Satoh, N. *et al.* Reaction of sevoflurane and its degradation products with soda lime. *Anesthesiology*, **77**, 1155–1164 (1992)

30. Frink, E. J., Malan, T. P., Morhan, S. E., Brown, E. A., Malcomson, M. and Brown, B. R. Quantification of the degradation products of sevoflurane in two CO_2 absorbants during low-flow anesthesia in surgical patients. *Anesthesiology*, **77**, 1064–1069 (1992)

31. Morgan, S. R., Frink, E. J., Kotake, Y., Malan, T. P. and Salmon, R. Evaluation of pulmonary injury from sevoflurane degradation products during closed circuit anesthesia in dogs. *Anesthesiology*, **79** (Suppl.), A409 (1993)

32. Bitoh, H. and Ikeda, K. Sevoflurane in closed circuit anesthesia. *Anesthesiology*, **75**, (Suppl.), A434 (1991)
33. Mazze, R. I. The safety of sevoflurane in humans. *Anesthesiology*, **77**, 1062–1063 (1992)
34. Ahnefeld, F. W., Kilian, J. and Friesdorf, W. Sicherheit und Instandhaltung medizinisch-technischer Geräte. *Anästh. Intensivmed.*, **22**, 291–308 (1981)
35. Müchler, H. C. Das technische Narkoserisiko. *Prakt. Anästh.*, **13**, 368–378 (1978)
36. Good, M. L. and Paulus, D. A. Equipment. In *Manual of Complications During Anesthesia* (ed. N. Gravenstein), J. B. Lippincott, Philadelphia (1991), pp. 83–120
37. Johnstone, R. E. Equipment malfunction. In *Complications in Anesthesiology* (eds F. K. Orkin, and L. H. Cooperman), J. B. Lippincott, Philadelphia (1983), pp. 639–645
38. Conway, C. M. Closed and low flow systems: Theoretical considerations. *Acta Anaesth. Belg.*, **35**, 257–263 (1984)
39. Schrieber, P. Anesthesia systems. In *North American Draeger Safety Guidelines*, Merchants Press, Boston (1985)
40. Schreiber, P. and Schreiber, J. M. *Electronic Surveillance during Anesthesia*, North American Draeger (1986)
41. Opderbecke, H. W. Ärztliche Sorgfaltspflicht bei der Narkoseführung mit reduziertem Frischgasflow. In *Alternative Methoden in der Anästhesie* (eds P. Lawin, H. van Aken and U. Schneider), INA-Schriftenreihe, Bd. 50, Thieme, Stuttgart (1985), pp. 49–52
42. Cullen, S. C. Who is watching the patient? *Anesthesiology*, **37**, 361–362 (1972)
43. Edsall, D. W. Economy is not the major benefit of closed-system anesthesia. *Anesthesiology*, **54**, 258 (1981)
44. Deshane, P. D. and Edsall, D. W. Incidence of hypoxemia due to a hypoxic mixture in low flow anesthesia when using nitrous oxide. Abstracts of the Annual Meeting of the Society for Technology in Anesthesia, *Human Performance and Anesthesia Technology*, 17–19 February 1993, New Orleans, p. 49
45. Eyrich, K. Sorgfalt bei der Prämedikation und Wahl des Anästhesieverfahrens. *Anästh. Intensivmed.*, **20**, 39–43 (1979)
46. Lotz, P. Sicherheitstechnische Aspekte bei der Anwendung medizinisch-technischer Geräte im Krankenhaus. *mt-Medizintechnik*, **104**, 133–137 (1984)
47. Lunn, J. N. and Mushin, W. W. *Mortality Associated with Anaesthesia*, Nuffield Provincial Hospitals Trust, London (1982)
48. Calkins, J. M. Why new delivery systems? In *Future Anesthesia Delivery Systems* (eds B. R. Brown, J. M. Calkins and R. J. Saunders), *Contemporary Anesthesia Practice*, Vol. VIII, Davies, Philadelphia (1984), pp. 3–9
49. Cooper, J. B., Newborner, R. S. and Kitz, R. J. An analysis of major errors and equipment failures in anesthesia management: considerations for prevention and detection. *Anesthesiology*, **60**, 34–42 (1984)
50. Keats, A. S. What do we know about anesthetic mortality? *Anesthesiology*, **50**, 387–392 (1979)
51. Opderbecke, H. W. Sorgfalt bei der Durchführung und Überwachung der Anästhesie. *Anästh. Intensivmed.*, **20**, 59–62 (1979)
52. Mazzia, V. D. B. and Simon, A. H. Low flow and close system anesthesia: legal liability and some specific cases. In *Low Flow and Closed System Anesthesia* (eds J. A. Aldrete, H. J. Lowe and R. W. Virtue), Grune and Stratton, New York (1979), pp. 315–321
53. Spieß, W. Minimal-flow Anästhesie – eine zeitgemäße Alternative für die Klinikroutine. *Anaesth. Reanim.*, **5**, 145–159 (1980)
54. Virtue, R. W. Toward closed system anesthesia. *Anaesthesist*, **26**, 545–546 (1977)
55. Ernst, E. A. and Spain, J. A. Closed-circuit and high-flow systems: examining alternatives. In *Future Anesthesia Delivery Systems* (eds B. R. Brown, J. M. Calkins and R. J. Saunders), *Contemporary Anesthesia Practice.*, Vol. VIII, F. A. Davies, Philadelphia (1984), pp. 11–38
56. Baum, J. and Strauß, J. M. Kohlenmonoxidbildung im Atemkalk. *Anästh. Intensivmed.*, **36**, 237–240 (1995)
57. Parker, C. R. J. and Snowdon, S. L. Predicted and measured oxygen concentrations in the circle system using low fresh gas flows with osygen supplied by an oxygen concentrator. *Br. J. Anaesth.*, **61**, 397–402 (1988)

10

Minimal flow anaesthesia in clinical practice

Minimal flow anaesthesia, as recommended by Virtue[1], is that low flow technique in which the fresh gas flow is reduced to the greatest possible extent if currently available anaesthetic equipment is used. It is the extreme form of anaesthesia with semi-closed rebreathing system, the breathing system on which the technical concept of most anaesthetic machines is based. Thus, minimal flow anaesthesia corresponds well to the defined range of operation of the apparatus. The safety facilities provided by different European and American standards and regulations comprehensively meet the requirements concerning the safety of patients. This chapter deals with the practical rules and recommendations for safe performance of minimal flow anaesthesia in clinical practice.

At first, low flow anaesthetic techniques should only be applied in uncomplicated surgical operations and on patients not suffering from critical disease. Thus, full attention can be paid to both the patient and the anaesthetic machine while gaining experience with the new technique. It ought to go without saying, yet it should be emphasized once more, that, in the case of high risk patients or surgical interventions, the anaesthetist must only employ a suitable anaesthetic method with which he is best acquainted. From the medicolegal aspect, however, minimal flow anaesthesia must be accepted as an anaesthetic technique appropriate for routine clinical use. Much scientific investigation has been dedicated to this method which thus can be considered to be an equal alternative to common anaesthetic practice. As early as 1986, Bergmann[2] pointed out that performance of anaesthesia with high fresh gas flow, as is most commonly employed, is in marked contrast to the high technical standards of modern anaesthetic machines.

10.1 Maintenance of the equipment

Following daily use, the breathing system, including all valves, is completely disassembled, cleaned, sterilized or disinfected in line with the respective instructions for use. It must be ensured that all sealing rings are removed from their grooves to be carefully cleaned. Thereafter, all components are dried and laid out for cooling.

If the breathing system is equipped with a switch, prior to reassembly of the cleaned components, the stopcock has to be lubricated with an oxygen-safe grease (e.g. Oxygenoex S4, Drägerwerk, Lübeck, Germany). The leakproofness required for minimal flow anaesthesia can only be achieved if brittle and hard seals are removed and all screw connections of the circle system are tightened carefully but not excessively. Plastic components of the system such as absorber canisters and valve domes have to be thoroughly checked for hairline cracks and replaced if necessary. Metal tapers have to be checked for damage, and cleanliness and correct fit of all metal-to-metal connections must be verified. This approach ensures that the required gas tightness of the breathing system with a leakage loss less than 100 ml/min at a pressure of 2 kPa ($\simeq 20$ cmH$_2$O) can always be achieved in routine clinical use. It is good practice to keep a small number of seals and plastic components available as spare parts.

Where the use of double absorbers is concerned, the contents of the absorber adjacent to the circle system should be discarded whenever the soda lime is exhausted, but it should be routinely replaced after at most one week's use. The same procedure should be adopted if single absorbers are used with continuous carbon dioxide monitoring. Bacteriological investigations in the present author's own department confirmed that this procedure can be considered to be very safe in terms of hygiene[3,4]. When the absorbent is discarded, the absorber canister should be disassembled as far as possible, and care should be taken again that rubber seals are removed from their grooves. The disassembled absorber has to be disinfected or sterilized in accordance with the manufacturer's instructions for use. After cleaning, the sealing rings and components are reassembled when they have cooled down to room temperature. When the clean absorber has been refilled, a label indicating the filling date is attached to the canister.

A patient hose system is attached to the circle system immediately after reassembly and the breathing system carefully tested for leaks. The APL valve at the circle absorber system has to be closed and the corrguated hoses attached to the Y-piece as shown in Figure 10.1. A high oxygen flow is then supplied to the system in order to build up a pressure of 2 kPa ($\simeq 20$ cmH$_2$O) within the system. Then the oxygen flow is reduced to 100 ml/min: under these conditions, the pressure of 2 kPa must not fall over a period of 1 min. In the author's department, the leak test is performed routinely at a pressure of 4 kPa ($\simeq 40$ cmH$_2$O), a tightness which can be achieved even in routine use of the anaesthetic machines if maintenance is conducted in the described manner.

Some anaesthetic machines will require specific procedures in leak tests; for instance in the AV 1 (Drägerwerk, Lübeck, Germany), the leak test has to be performed as follows: the manual bag is detached from its corrugated hose and the hose is then attached to the Y-piece for connection with the patient system as illustrated in Figure 10.1. The ventilation mode switch is set to the MAN (FLOW +) function, and the APL valve to its maximum opening pressure of 8 kPa ($\simeq 80$ cmH$_2$O). By control of the fine needle valve, oxygen is fed into the system to build up a pressure of 4 kPa ($\simeq 40$ cmH$_2$O). Once this pressure is gained, the oxygen supply into the system is stopped. If the pressure does not drop below 2.5 kPa ($\simeq 25$ cmH$_2$O) within 1 min, the system will be sufficiently tight for performance of minimal flow anaesthesia. If the pressure drops from 4 to 3 kPa ($\simeq 40$–30 cmH$_2$O) within a period of 15 s, this corresponds to a leakage rate of 250 ml/min.

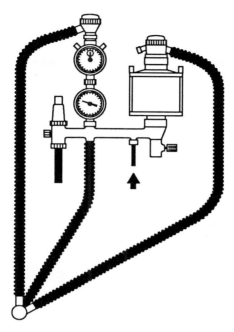

Figure 10.1   Connections of hose assembly for performance of leak test: circle absorption system 8 ISO (Drägerwerk, Lübeck, Germany)

The breathing systems of the Cato, Cicero and Cicero EM (Drägerwerk, Lübeck, Germany) and EAS 9010, EAS 9020 and Elsa (Gambro-Engström, Bromma, Sweden) anaesthetic machines are tested for leaks in a test sequence which is run automatically (see Section 7.2.4.1). After having passed the check successfully, the gas tightness of the breathing system and the ventilator will meet the requirements for performance of each kind of low flow anaesthesia, even with the lowest fresh gas flows.

Testing of other individual units of the cleaned machine is carried out in line with the respective instructions for use.

Proper function of all monitoring systems has to be verified at the beginning of each working day. This includes, if required, calibration and zero adjustment of the gas analyser and calibration of the oxygen monitor to 21% O_2 with ambient air. Furthermore, readiness for use of the anaesthetic machine and gas tightness of the breathing system must be tested every day prior to the start of the first anaesthetic.

10.1.1   Are there greater demands on disinfection or sterilization of the equipment resulting from fresh gas flow reduction?

In minimal flow anaesthesia the temperature and the humidity of the anaesthetic gases increase significantly. As increased warmth and humidity facilitates bacterial growth in the event of contamination, the question may

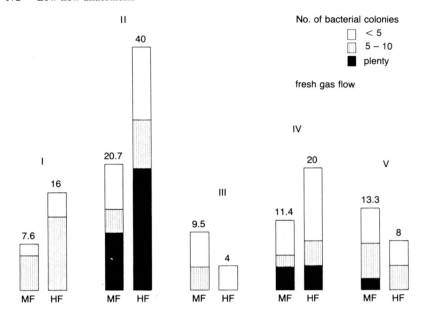

Figure 10.2   Percentage of positive bacteriological samples, related to the total number of samples taken at the corresponding sample site I–V. Comparison between the high flow (HF) and the minimal flow (MF) group. I, Connection between expired hose and expired valve; II, connection between manual bag and breathing system; III, taper at the expired side of the CO_2 absorber; IV, taper at the inspired side of the CO_2 absorber; V, connection between inspired hose and inspired valve (From Baum[3])

be raised whether routine performance of minimal flow anaesthesia increases the risk of bacterial contamination of the breathing system.

In the author's investigation[3] of this topic, 546 bacteriological samples were taken with the aid of cotton-tipped swabs at different sites in the breathing system, 55 (14%) of them showing bacterial contamination. Twenty-one (38%) of the 55 positive results were found at the point where the manual bag is attached to the anaesthetic circuit with a rubber hose (sampling site II). At the other sampling sites, only minor bacterial contamination was found. Even if the results were differentiated according to the number of bacterial colonies, the highest incidence of plentiful colonies could be found at this particular sampling site II.

With two anaesthetic machines, minimal flow anaesthesia was performed routinely, while with another anaesthetic apparatus, anaesthesia with high fresh gas flow was carried out exclusively. If the results were differentiated according to the fresh gas flow used, a statistical difference could not be established between the two groups (Figure 10.2). There is thus no evidence of an increase of bacterial contamination caused by flow reduction. These results correspond with the findings of Bengtson et al.[5].

The investigation was performed under the following conditions. According to the rules given by the German Society for Anaesthesia and Intensive Care Medicine DGAI[6], the masks, the Y-pieces and the corrugated patient hoses were changed with every patient, parts of the breathing system were disinfected on a daily schedule, and all parts of the circuit were sterilized weekly. As the manual bag with its connecting tube was considered to be a part of the circuit itself, it was only changed and disinfected weekly. The results of the investigation suggest that the manual bag and the connecting rubber tube should also preferably to be changed on a daily basis. The site where the rubber hose is connected to the circuit seems to be a favoured location for bacterial growth. Generally, this is the lowest point of the breathing circle where accumulation of condensed water is likely, thus facilitating the growth of microbes, such as *Pseudomonas*, which prefer a warm and humid environment.

The following recommendations seem to be justified by these results:

- the routine performance of anaesthesia with reduced fresh gas flow does not increase the risk of bacterial contamination of the breathing system if cleaning and sterilization procedures are accomplished properly
- bacterial contamination, however, seems to increase if a previously used breathing system is left un-utilized without cleaning for a period of time
- there is absolutely no evidence that there is an aerogenic spread of bacterial contamination by the gas flow either in the high flow or the low flow group
- care should be taken to change the manual bag with its connecting hose on a daily schedule
- in addition, the author recommends not attaching the manual bag to the circuit prior to its next use, but leaving the adapter open, thus allowing adequate drying of the metal-to-rubber connection
- as most of the identified bacterial strains are common skin commensals, the hands should be disinfected before reassembling the circuit after cleaning and sterilizing; furthermore, disinfection of the hands should be obligatory whenever the patient hoses are changed after use.

Whether the use of bacterial filters offers real advantages in preventing cross-contamination by anaesthetic equipment has long been controversial[7]. One must agree with the logical hypothesis that bacterial filters reduce contamination of the equipment[8], but Luttropp admits that their absence does not increase contamination either of the circle or the ventilator. If, however, anaesthetic equipment and ventilators are decontaminated daily to minimize the risk of cross-infection, the use of bacterial filters is obviously unnecessary. Whether the use of bacterial filters really reduces the water content of the anaesthetic gas circulating in the breathing system in low flow anaesthesia[8] has not yet been verified. The use of filters as heat and moisture exchangers (HME) to ensure adequate humidification and warming of the anaesthetic gases is also judged to be unnecessary if anaesthesia is performed with a rebreathing system[9], especially if low flow techniques are applied (see Section 6.4).

10.2   Fresh gas composition

The fresh gas composition of 60% oxygen and 40% nitrous oxide, as recommended by Virtue, guarantees a sufficiently high inspired oxygen concentration. During the first 60 min after flow reduction it rises to an average of 38% (Figure 10.3). These figures are very close to those quoted by Virtue himself and the nitrous oxide concentration is correspondingly low.

If the fresh gas composition is set to 50% oxygen and 50% nitrous oxide for a more effective utilization of the nitrous oxide and to achieve a concentration resulting in significant analgesia and amnesia[10-12], the inspired oxygen concentration drops to a value of 28% during the first 60 min in 30% of all cases (Figure 10.4a,b). As an inspired oxygen concentration of at least 30% is recommended to reliably prevent accidental hypoxaemia[10,13], the fresh gas composition must be modified in favour of oxygen whenever the lower alarm limit of 28% is reached: the oxygen flow is increased by 50 ml/min and the nitrous oxide flow decreased by the same value (Figure 10.5). This holds for any of the low flow techniques: whenever the inspired oxygen concentration drops to the lower limit, the oxygen flow must be increased by 10% of the total fresh gas flow and the nitrous oxide flow has to be reduced by the same amount.

More detailed investigation shows that, particularly in heavyweight, athletic and young patients, the inspired oxygen concentration drops to a distinctly greater extent to the given limit of 28% (Figure 10.6). These patient characteristics correlate well with an increased oxygen consumption. The higher the oxygen consumption, the higher the oxygen extraction from the alveolar gas. This correspondingly decreases the oxygen content of the rebreathing volume which, mixed with the given fresh gas volume, is returned to the patient in the following breaths[14].

During the early stages of learning this anaesthetic technique, it is advisable to adhere to the concept recommended by Virtue and to select a fresh gas

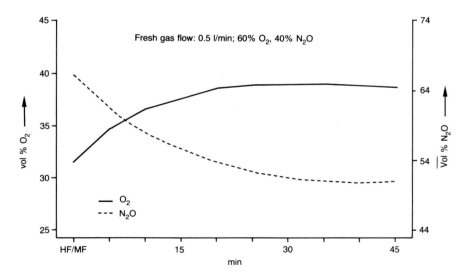

Figure 10.3 Alterations of the nitrous oxide and the oxygen concentration during the course of minimal flow anaesthesia. Fresh gas composition in accordance with the scheme given by Virtue[1]. HF/MF, time of flow reduction from 4.4 to 0.5 l/min

composition of 60% oxygen and 40% nitrous oxide at the point of flow reduction. Proceeding in this way, accidental hypoxia will be safely prevented. It must be borne in mind that, while oxygen consumption is virtually constant, corresponding to the basal metabolism[16], the nitrous oxide uptake decreases according to an exponential function during the course of anaesthesia[17].

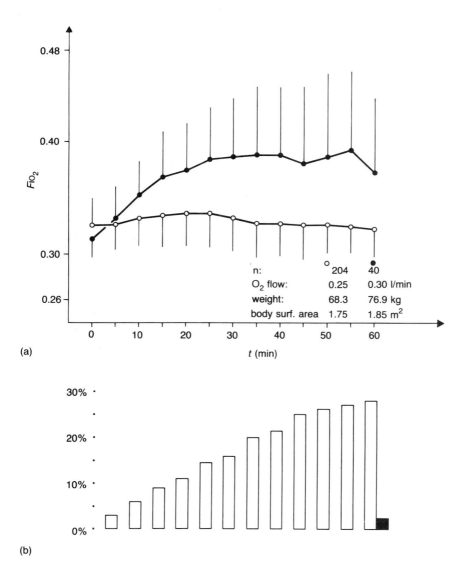

(a)

(b)

Figure 10.4 (a) Alterations of the inspired oxygen concentration (F_{IO_2}) during the course of minimal flow anaesthesia as a function of fresh gas composition: fresh gas flow 0.5 l/min–0.25 l/min O_2 and 0.25 l/min N_2O versus fresh gas flow 0.5 l/min–0.3 l/min O_2 and 0.2 l/min N_2O. Ordinate: F_{IO_2}, mean values and standard deviation; abscissa: time, starting with flow reduction. (b) Cumulative presentation of the relative frequency at which F_{IO_2} drops below the value of 0.28

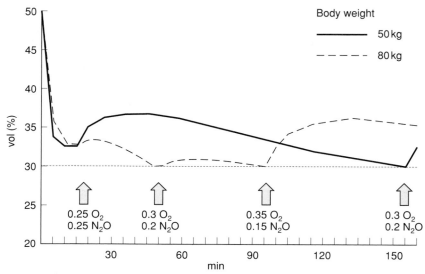

Figure 10.5 Inspired oxygen concentration during the course of minimal flow anaesthesia as a function of body weight (correlates to the oxygen uptake). At flow reduction, oxygen and nitrous oxide flow are set to 0.25 l/min each. Whenever the concentration drops to 30%, oxygen flow is increased by 0.05 l/min and nitrous oxide flow decreased by the same value (From Baum[15])

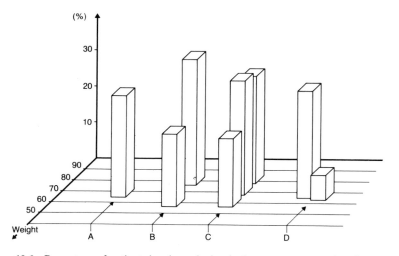

Figure 10.6 Percentage of patients in whom the inspired oxygen concentration drops to a value of 28%, as a function of patient weight, constitution and age: y-axis, percentage of patients (%); z-axis, body weight (kg).

A, Whole group of patients: average weight 69 kg, average age 41.5 years. Differentiated according to:
B. Body weight: average weight 59 kg versus average weight 78 kg
C, Constitution in accordance with the Broca index: underweight (average weight 58 kg) versus normal weight (average weight 67 kg) versus adipose patients (average weight 79 kg)
D, Age: average age 38 years versus average age 62 years (with virtually identical weight and stature).

Following flow reduction 15 min after induction, the volume of nitrous oxide initially being extracted from the system is greater than that supplied, so that the nitrous oxide concentration decreases while that of the oxygen increases correspondingly. However, about 35–45 min later, the nitrous oxide volume taken up by the patient becomes less than that fed into the system with the continuous flow of fresh gas. From now on the nitrous oxide concentration slowly increases as a result of nitrous oxide accumulation, whereas the oxygen concentration simultaneously tends to decrease. Even though the fresh gas composition has been adjusted as recommended by Virtue, it must be expected that, in the case of long surgical interventions, the inspired oxygen concentration drops to values below 30%. In this case, the fresh gas composition has to be modified in favour of oxygen.

In addition, it has to be emphasized that the adjustment of conventional needle valves in the range of 10–20 ml/min cannot be guaranteed, not even by very careful equipment handling. Since the precision of flowmeters is quoted as being ±10% of the set value, the total deviation of the oxygen and nitrous oxide flow may finally amount to about 50 ml/min. It is for this reason that minimal flow anaesthesia may on no account be performed without continuous measurement of the inspired oxygen concentration. Furthermore, the lower alarm limit of the monitoring device should be set carefully to 28–30%. Whenever the oxygen concentration drops to this limit, the oxygen flow has to be increased by 50 ml/min and the nitrous oxide flow reduced accordingly.

10.3   Administration of volatile anaesthetics

10.3.1   Isoflurane

In addition to the volatile anaesthetics halothane and enflurane, the latter's stereoisomer, isoflurane, has been available for clinical use since 1981.

Due to its specific physicochemical and pharmacological properties, isoflurane is particularly suited to performance of minimal flow anaesthesia (Table 10.1). Fast wash-in and wash-out of the anaesthetic can be expected because of its low solubility in blood. The anaesthetic depth required for performance of surgical interventions can be reached rapidly because of its

Table 10.1   Physicochemical and pharmacological properties of inhalational anaesthetics (After references 18, 19 and 22–25)*

	MAC	$\lambda_{B/G}$	$\lambda_{Oil/gas}$	VAP	Mol. wt	MR
Nitrous oxide	101	0.47	1.4	—	44.02	0.004%
Halothane	0.77	2.3	224	226	197.4	20–30%
Enflurane	1.68	1.78	96.5	198	184.5	2–7%
Isoflurane	1.15	1.41	90.8	194	184.5	0.2–1%
Sevoflurane	2.0	0.65	42	183	200.1	3–7%
Desflurane	$\simeq$4–6	0.42	18	209	168.0	<0.2%
Xenon	71	0.14	1.9	—	131.3	0%

*MAC, minimum alveolar concentration; $\lambda_{B/G}$, blood/gas partition coefficient; $\lambda_{oil/gas}$, oil/gas partition coefficient; VAP, ml vapour/ml fluid of the volatile anaesthetic at 20°C; Mol. wt, molecular weight; MR, metabolic rate.

low minimum alveolar concentration (MAC)[18,19]. Its metabolism at about 0.2% is extremely low[20], so that the uptake is not thereby increased. The amount of agent, calculated in accordance with Lowe's uptake formula (see Section 3.3.1.2), which has to be supplied to the patient for maintenance of a defined expired concentration, is lower than is the case for halothane or enflurane. A simple and easily manageable standardized dosage scheme has been developed for isoflurane which considerably improves the practicability of minimal flow anaesthesia[21].

During an initial phase of 15–20 min using high fresh gas flow (4.4 l/min), the fresh gas isoflurane concentration may be uniformly set to 1.5%. After reduction of the fresh gas flow to 0.5 l/min, the concentration is increased to

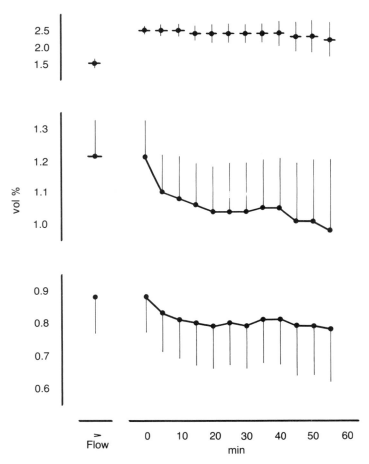

Figure 10.7   Inspired and expired isoflurane concentration immediately prior to, and during the course of 60 min after flow reduction to 0.5 l/min (mean values and standard deviation). Group of patients: average weight 74 kg, average age 51 years. Upper ordinate: vaporizer setting = fresh gas concentration; centre ordinate: inspired isoflurane concentration; bottom ordinate, expired isoflurane concentration. Measuring device: Normac (Datex, Helsinki, Finland)

a standard value of 2.5%. Modifications of this scheme have to be made in accordance with the requirements of the surgical intervention or the individual reaction of the patient, as would be the case during high flow isoflurane anaesthesia.

Applying this standardized dosage scheme results in an average expired and thus approximately alveolar isoflurane concentration of 0.8%, i.e. about 0.7 MAC (Figure 10.7). If the MAC share of 0.6, due to a nitrous oxide concentration of 55–65%, is added to this value[26], a common MAC value of 1.3 is achieved. This is the anaesthetic alveolar concentration at which 95% of all patients do not react to the skin incision (AD_{95}). The expired isoflurane concentration of 0.8% is achieved virtually independent of patient characteristics such as weight, constitution and age (Figure 10.8–10.10).

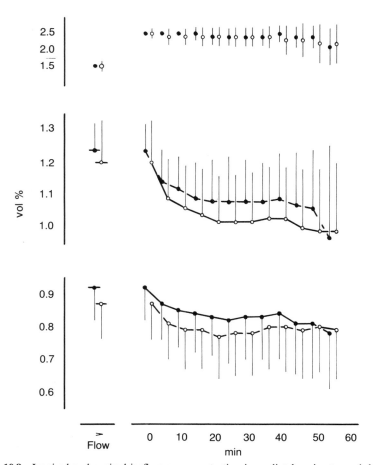

Figure 10.8 Inspired and expired isoflurane concentration immediately prior to, and during the course of 60 min after flow reduction to 0.5 l/min (mean values and standard deviation). Differentiation of the whole group (see Figure 10.7) according to body weight: ● average weight 62 kg (average age 49 years) versus ○ average weight 81 kg (average age 52 years). Upper ordinate, vaporizer setting = fresh gas concentration; centre ordinate, inspired isoflurane concentration; bottom ordinate, expired isoflurane concentration

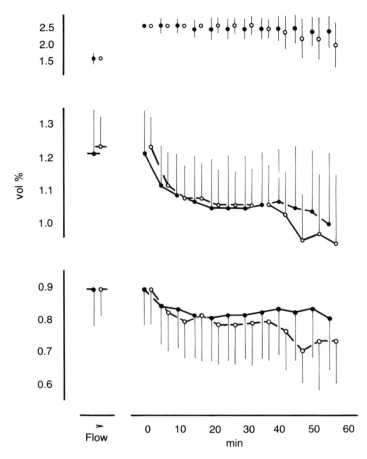

Figure 10.9   Inspired and expired isoflurane concentration immediately prior to, and during the course of 60 min after flow reduction to 0.5 l/min (mean values and standard deviation). Differentiation of the whole group (see Figure 10.7) according to age: ● average age 46 years (average weight 75 kg) versus ○ average age 69 years (average weight 74 kg). Upper ordinate, vaporizer setting = fresh gas concentration; centre ordinate, inspired isoflurane concentration; bottom ordinate, expired isoflurane concentration

It must be pointed out, however, that the MAC varies with a number of individual factors such as age, body temperature and, furthermore, with variations of anaesthetic management, such as supplementary analgesics and premedicants[20,27]. Furthermore, the pharmacokinetics of a volatile anaesthetic vary as a function of individual parameters such as age and cardiac output[20,26,27]. Although quotations for patients' average values can be made with sufficient accuracy with respect to inspired and expired isoflurane concentration if this dosage scheme is applied, in the individual case the concentration may differ considerably from these predicted values. In addition, it must be emphasized that only a certain gas concentration is

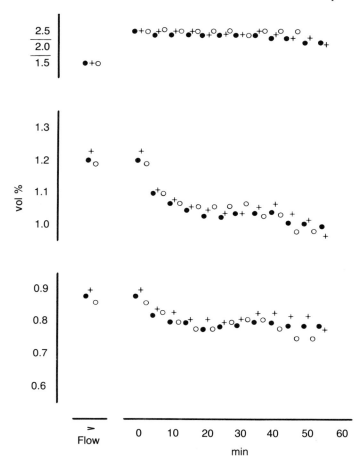

Figure 10.10   Inspired and expired isoflurane concentration immediately prior to, and during the course of 60 min after flow reduction to 0.5 l/min (mean values and standard deviation). Differentiation of the group (see Figure 10.7) according to constitution: ● adipose (average weight 81 kg, average age 53 years) versus ○ underweight (average weight 56, average age 37 years) versus + normal weight patients (average weight 67 kg, average age 49 years). Upper ordinate, vaporizer setting = fresh gas concentration; centre ordinate, inspired isoflurane concentration; bottom ordinate, expired isoflurane concentration

predicted with this dosage scheme. It is not possible, however, to predict precisely whether the anaesthetic depth achieved with this concentration will meet the demands of the specific surgical intervention or the individual status of the patient. Based on the standard scheme of the anaesthetic fresh gas concentration, further adjustment of the agent concentration has to be made in the light of current clinical requirements, as is the case with high flow anaesthesia.

The standardized dosage scheme for isoflurane has proved its worth outstandingly in clinical practice. This confirms Lin's thesis (see Section 3.3.1.4) that, following an initial phase of anaesthesia during which the gas concentrations within the whole system are brought to equilibrium, the uptake of volatile anaesthetics remains relatively constant. Assuming stable cardiac output and unaltered ventilation, it is essentially a function of the alveolar–capillary partial pressure difference. Lin therefore recommends replacing the low uptake loss by administering comparatively low anaesthetic concentrations, which can be kept constant over a long period of time. He suggests that involved calculations and frequent changes in vapour settings in accordance with a complex exponential function are unnecessary.

Following on from Lin's quotations on halothane and enflurane, the following formula can be used for calculation of isoflurane dosage. After an initial equilibrium phase, the uptake for the following 60 min can be estimated by means of the formula

$$\text{Uptake}_{\text{iso}} = 10\text{–}15\,\text{ml isoflurane vapour per \% desired concentration}$$

10.3.2   Enflurane

According to the Lin concept, the dosage guidelines can also be simplified to improve the practicability of minimal flow anaesthesia if enflurane is used as volatile anaesthetic. During the initial 15–20 min phase of anaesthesia with a high fresh gas flow (4.4 l/min), a fresh gas concentration of 2.5% enflurane results in an average expired concentration of 1.35%. If a uniform fresh gas concentration of 3.5% is set at the time that the flow is reduced to 0.5 l/min, the expired concentration drops to an average of 0.95% within the next 30 min. It is thus only a little lower than the desired value of 1.1% which corresponds to $0.65 \times \text{MAC}_{\text{enf}}$. Additional to the MAC_{N2O} of about 0.65, this results in a common value of $1.3 \times \text{MAC}$, corresponding again to the AD_{95}, the anaesthetic concentration which ensures sufficient anaesthetic depth for skin incision in 95% of all patients (Figure 10.11).

If patients are studied according to body weight, the concentration gained in low weight patients is altogether higher than that in heavyweight patients (Figure 10.12).

The following conclusion can be drawn from clinical experience with this standardized scheme for enflurane dosage in minimal flow anaesthesia. It is perfectly possible to obtain good clinical results by standardization of enflurane dosage without using an involved time-dependent scheme. However, equilibrium processes during minimal flow anaesthesia proceed slower than those with isoflurane. The inspired and expired concentrations depend to a distinctly greater extent on patient characteristics such as weight and constitution.

10.3.3   Halothane

The first experiences gained in the performance of minimal flow anaesthesia with halothane and guidelines for its use in anaesthesia with maximum flow reduction were published as early as 1959 by Robson et al.[28].

A dosage concept for halothane will only be mentioned in order to complete the discussion. Where adults are concerned, compared with enflurane and isoflurane, its use is viewed rather critically because of the potential hepatotoxic side-effects[29–31] and the aforementioned degradation of this

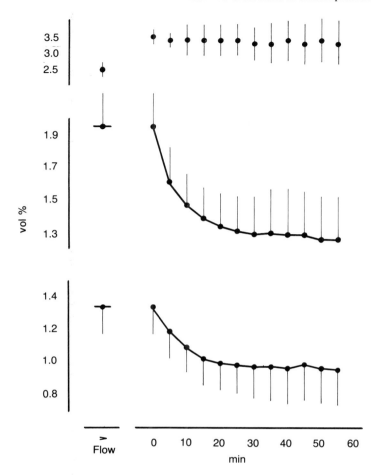

Figure 10.11   Inspired and expired enflurane concentration immediately prior to, and during the course of 60 min after flow reduction to 0.5 l/min (mean values and standard deviation). Group of patients: average weight 71 kg, average age 42 years. Upper ordinate, vaporizer setting = fresh gas concentration; centre ordinate, inspired enflurane concentration; bottom ordinate, expired enflurane concentration

agent with soda lime (see Section 9.1.2.2.7). As this volatile anaesthetic has not been used for several years in the present author's department, the clinical application of the concept was based on computer simulation of a halothane anaesthetic (see Chapter 5). In the initial phase of anaesthesia, the fresh gas halothane concentration was standardized at 2.0%, and to 4.0% after flow reduction.

During the initial high flow phase the average expired concentration amounts to 0.93%, decreases to 0.8% within 15 min after fresh gas flow reduction and tends to rise distinctly during the following course of anaesthesia (Figure 10.13). These values are distinctly above the desired

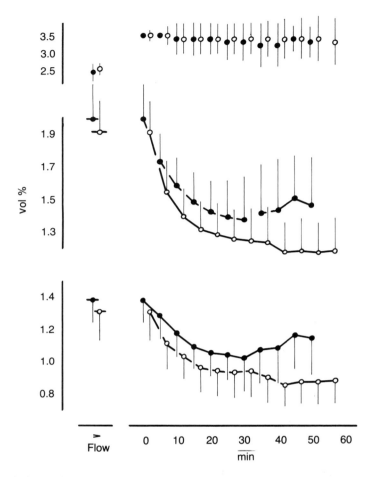

Figure 10.12 Inspired and expired enflurane concentration immediately prior to, and during the course of 60 min after flow reduction to 0.5 l/min (mean values and standard deviation). Differentiation of the group (see Figure 10.11) according to body weight: ● average weight 62 kg (average age 39 years) versus ○ average weight 79 kg (average age 44 years). Upper ordinate, vaporizer setting = fresh gas concentration; centre ordinate, inspired enflurane concentration; bottom ordinate, expired enflurane concentration.

concentration of $0.65 \times \text{MAC}_{\text{HAL}}$ (about 0.5% halothane). Clinical impressions also indicate an anaesthetic level somewhat too deep for most of the patients. Again, if patients are grouped according to body weight, there are pronounced differences in the resultant inspired and expired concentrations (Figure 10.14). If, in spite of the problems mentioned, halothane is used in a standardized dosage concept, a lower fresh gas concentration of about 3% to 2.5% has to be set at the vaporizer after flow reduction to 0.5 l/min (Figure 10.15). In the individual case, it must be expected that the values obtained in clinical practice may differ considerably from the quoted average values.

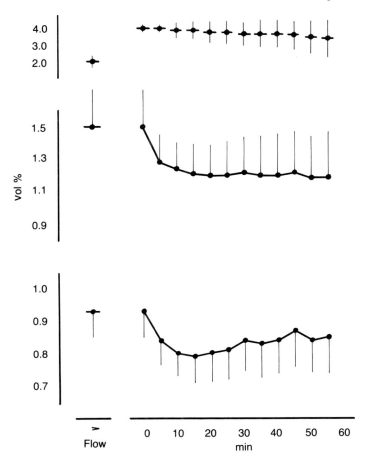

Figure 10.13   Inspired and expired halothane concentration immediately prior to, and during the course of 60 min after flow reduction to 0.5 l/min (mean values and standard deviation). Group of patients: average weight 72 kg, average age 41 years. Upper ordinate, vaporizer setting = fresh gas concentration; centre ordinate, inspired halothane concentration; bottom ordinate, expired halothane concentration

10.4   Concept and practical advice on performance of minimal flow anaesthesia with isoflurane

Isoflurane is ideally suited for use in minimal flow anaesthesia, which must be attributed to its favourable physicochemical and pharmacological properties. If the standardized dosage scheme is applied, it is possible to achieve a desired anaesthetic concentration, virtually independently of individual characteristics such as weight, constitution and age. The resultant anaesthetic depth is sufficient for most surgical interventions. Further instructions on dosage are not necessary as alterations in the anaesthetic fresh gas concentration have to be made according to clinical requirements.

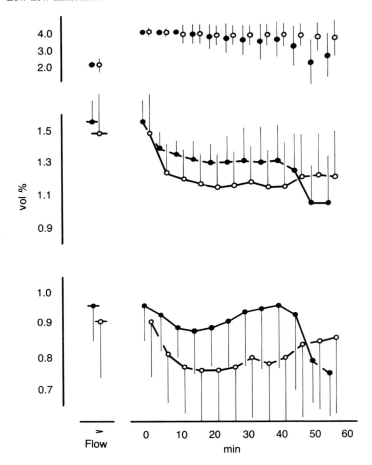

Figure 10.14 Inspired and expired halothane concentration immediately prior to, and during the course of 60 min after flow reduction to 0.5 l/min (mean values and standard deviation). Differentiation of the group (see Figure 10.13) according to body weight: ● average weight 57 kg (average age 38 years) versus ○ average weight 78 kg (average age 42 years). Upper ordinate, vaporizer setting = fresh gas concentration; centre ordinate, inspired halothane concentration; bottom ordinate, expired halothane concentration

Performance of minimal flow anaesthesia with isoflurane thus corresponds to the familiar procedure of anaesthesia with high fresh gas flows, which greatly improves the practicability of the method.

The following is a detailed description of the concept for minimal flow anaesthesia with isoflurane as is routinely practised in the author's department (Table 10.2).

Premedication is by means of intramuscular injection of atropine 0.01 mg/kg and midazolam 0.1 mg/kg, 45 min prior to the start of anaesthesia. Other schemes may be used according to the choice of the anaesthetist.

Following pre-curarization with a non-depolarizing muscle relaxant, anaesthesia is induced with thiopentone 3–5 mg/kg or etomidate 0.2 mg/kg,

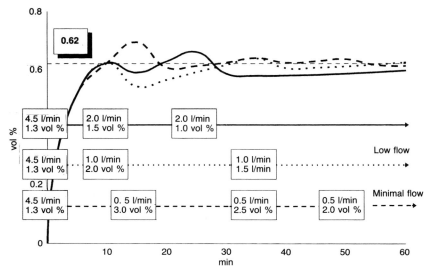

Figure 10.15   Expired halothane concentration (desired nominal value $0.62\% \equiv 0.8$ MAC) resulting from different vaporizer settings at different fresh gas flows. Assumed patient body weight: 75 kg (From Baum[15])

Table 10.2   Standardized concept for performance of minimal flow anaesthesia

Premedication
According to usual premedication scheme

Induction of anaesthesia
Preoxygenation
Intravenous hypnotic
Relaxation and intubation or insertion of a laryngeal mask
Connection to the circle absorber system

Initial phase of anaesthesia
Duration about 15–20 min
1.4 l/min oxygen
3.0 l/min nitrous oxide
Setting of the vaporizer
  isoflurane 1.0–1.5%
  enflurane 2.0–2.5%
  halothane 1.0–1.3%

Monitoring
Lower alarm limit insp. oxygen: 28–30%
Disconnection alarm: 5 cmH$_2$O below peak pressure
Expired minute volume: 0.5 l/min below nominal value
Upper alarm limit insp. volatile anaesthetic concentration: 2.0–2.5%

Fresh gas flow reduction
0.25–0.3 l/min oxygen
0.25–0.2 l/min nitrous oxide
Setting of the vaporizer
  isoflurane 2.5%
  enflurane 3.5%
  halothane 2.5–3.0%   *continued*

Table 10.2   *Continued*

Alteration of the fresh gas composition

Inspired oxygen concentration drops to lower limit
Oxygen flow is increased by 0.05 l/min
Nitrous oxide flow is decreased by 0.05 l/min

Volatile anaesthetic concentration needs to be increased (*maintaining long time constant*)
Fresh gas flow maintained at 0.5 l/min
Vaporizer's setting is increased by 1–2%
After achievement of the aspired new nominal value, reduction of the vaporizer setting: 0.5% higher than the starting point

Volatile anaesthetic concentration needs to be decreased (*maintaining long time constant*)
Fresh gas flow maintained at 0.5 l/min
Vaporizer's setting is decreased by 1–3.5%
After achievement of the desired new nominal value, vaporizer is set to 1–2%

Volatile anaesthetic concentration needs to be changed rapidly (*changing from long to short time constant*)
Vaporizer is set to the aspired nominal value
Fresh gas flow is increased to 4.4 l/min (1.4 l/min O$_2$, 3.0 l/min N$_2$O)
After achievement of the desired nominal value (usually about 5 min): low fresh gas flow is re-established at 0.5 l/min (0.3 l/min O$_2$, 0.2 l/min N$_2$O)
Vaporizer is set to a value 0.5% higher or 1–2% lower, respectively, than the starting point
Alternatively, anaesthetic depth may be increased rapidly by an intravenous injection of a supplementary hypnotic or analgesic drug

Gas volume deficiency; peak pressure and minute volume decrease
Replenishing the anaesthetic gas reservoir by short-term increase of the fresh gas flow
Search for leaks
In case of continuing leakage loss: increase of the fresh gas flow by 0.5 l/min and switch to low flow anaesthesia

Emergence from anaesthesia
Vaporizer is switched off 15–30 min prior to termination of the surgical intervention
Fresh gas flow is maintained at 0.5 l/min
Assist patient to spontaneous breathing
Flush system with 5 l/min oxygen 5–10 min prior to extubation
Postoperative care according to usual scheme

---

supplemented by fentanyl 0.1–0.2 mg if required. The patient is intubated after about 2 min of preoxygenation by ventilation with 5 l/min pure oxygen via a face mask and muscle relaxation.

A fresh gas flow of 4.4 l/min (1.4 l/min) O$_2$, 3.0 l/min N$_2$O) with an isoflurane concentration of 1.5% is set in the initial phase of anaesthesia using a circle absorber system. Additive muscle relaxant is given according to the clinical needs. Controlled ventilation is started as soon as possible. The high fresh gas flow is maintained over the following 15–20 min. During this period, nitrogen is washed out of the system, the gas concentrations brought to equilibrium within the entire gas-carrying space and thus the anaesthetic level deepened in a sufficiently short period of time.

The utmost care has to be taken that the alarm functions of all monitors are activated as soon as the patient is connected to the anaesthetic machine. The lower alarm limit at the oxygen monitor is set to 28–30%, the disconnection alarm adjusted to a value 0.5 kPa ($\simeq 5$ cmH$_2$O) below the peak pressure, the occlusion alarm to 3 kPa ($\simeq 30$ cmH$_2$O), and the upper alarm limit for the inspired aesthetic concentration to 2.0–2.5%, regardless of the agent used.

After completion of the initial high flow phase, the fresh gas flow is reduced to 0.5 l/min, at which point the oxygen concentration must be increased to at least 50%, but preferably to 60%. The setting of the isoflurane vaporizer has to be increased to 2.5%.

During the first 30 min after flow reduction, the patient still takes up a comparatively large volume of gas which is close to the fresh gas volume being supplied to the breathing system. In the event of very high uptake or additional gas loss via leaks, this early phase after flow reduction is the most prone to the development of gas volume deficiency.

Where conventional anaesthetic machines without gas reservoir and continuous fresh gas flow are concerned, this will result in insufficient expired filling of the ventilator, a decrease of tidal volume and of the peak pressure. Given careful adjustment of the alarms, this problem will be recognized immediately. If anaesthetic ventilators are used with hanging bellows which are expanded actively during expiration, the ventilatory pattern may change from intermittent positive pressure ventilation (IPPV) to alternating pressure ventilation (APV). In this case, too, proper adjustment of the alarms will ensure immediate identification of the problem.

In the event of gas volume deficiency, the fresh gas flow has to be increased for adequate supply of gas volume to the breathing system and the ventilator, thus replenishing the volume shortage. When sufficient filling of the system is restored again, the leaks have to be detected and eliminated. If the morning leak test of the system has been carried out correctly, losses are in most cases caused by leaks at the joint between patient hose assembly and the tube connector or an inadequate inflation of the cuff.

In this context, attention must be drawn to two potential sources of leaks. In accordance with obligatory regulations in Germany, all corrugated hoses are fitted with ISO connectors made of hard plastic. The connection between the rubber hose and the plastic connector loosens gradually following frequent heat disinfecting processes. The plastic connectors can then be quite easily rotated at the junction to the corrugated hose. The looser this connection, the greater the leakage loss at this point. The ISO-CLIC connector at the microbial filter (Drägerwerk, Lübeck, Germany) is also subject to ageing toward the end of the re-sterilization cycles. Apart from rare leaks at the filter housing, it can be frequently observed that the connection to the breathing system is loosening, which cannot be compensated for by the sealing ring supplied. In searching for leaks, it is therefore essential to consider such weak points.

If anaesthesia is performed with anaesthetic machines which feature an anaesthetic gas reservoir and discontinuous supply of the fresh gas into the breathing system (AV 1, Cato, Cicero, Megamed 700), the manual bag, which serves as the reservoir, should not be hung up at the machine by its rubber lug, but rather deposited freely on the trolley. Otherwise it is possible that the reservoir's gas volume may be drained by the tension caused by the weight of the connecting corrugated hose whenever the excess gas discharge valve opens during expiration. Smaller imbalances between the gas volume being lost by uptake and leaks and the volume being supplied to the breathing system will be evened out by the reservoir's volume. Only if the manual bag is emptied completely does the tidal volume tend to decrease. Thus a gas reservoir considerably facilitates the performance of anaesthesia with reduced fresh gas flows. The same applies for all anaesthetic machines in which the ventilator's volume itself serves as an anaesthetic gas reservoir. These are the ventilators with floating standing bellows (Servo Anesthesia System, Modulus CD, Excel) or the classical bag-in-bottle ventilators (EAS 9010 and 9020, Elsa, Ventilator 711). Only if the expiratory filling of the bag falls below the preset tidal volume does gas volume imbalance result in alteration of ventilation.

Shortage in gas volume resulting from high oxygen and nitrous oxide uptake may also necessitate intermittent short-term increase of the fresh gas flow in individual cases. Experience has shown, however, that within a period of 30 min after flow reduction and with further decrease of nitrous oxide uptake, the filling status of the system remains adequately stable in most cases. Otherwise the anaesthetist should switch to a total fresh gas flow of 0.7 l/min (0.35 l/min O_2, 0.35 l/min N_2O).

Similar to the procedure in high flow anaesthesia, isoflurane dosage during the course of anaesthesia is adjusted according to the clinical signs of anaesthetic depth. In a considerable number of cases the isoflurane concentration of the fresh gas must be reduced to 1.5–2.0% after about 45–120 min.

Due to the long time constant, in low flow anaesthesia all alterations of the anaesthetic fresh gas concentration become effective in the breathing system only with a considerable time delay. In the case of a rapidly required change of the anaesthetic level, two alternative ways to proceed are possible. While maintaining low fresh gas flow, rapid increase of anaesthetic depth can be accomplished by intravenous application of supplementary doses of fentanyl or thiopental (anaesthesia management maintaining a long time constant). However, if the change in anaesthetic depth is to be achieved by an increase in volatile agent concentration, the fresh gas flow has to be increased and its anaesthetic concentration adapted to the desired nominal value (anaesthesia management by changing the time constant). A rapid decrease of the anaesthetic depth always requires an increase of the fresh gas flow and appropriate adaptation of the vaporizer setting to achieve a lower anaesthetic concentration sufficiently fast (anaesthesia management with short time constant). If the fresh gas flow is increased to about 4 l/min to facilitate the wash-in of a desired volatile anaesthetic concentration, after a period of about 5 min the new nominal value will be gained. The flow can again be reduced, but care must be taken to again adapt the fresh gas composition according to the low flow conditions (Figures 10.16a and 10.16b).

If the inspired oxygen concentration drops to the lower limit of 30% O_2, the oxygen flow has to be increased by 0.05 l/min while nitrous oxide is reduced by 0.05 l/min at the same time.

Where anaesthetic machines in which the manual bag is directly connected to the breathing system are concerned, a switch from mechanical to manual ventilation should only be performed at the end of the inspiratory phase. Otherwise, a considerable proportion of the total gas volume remains in the ventilator bellows, and the remaining volume circulating in the breathing system becomes too low for adequate ventilation. It is for the same reason that, when a switch is made from manual to mechanical ventilation, the gas

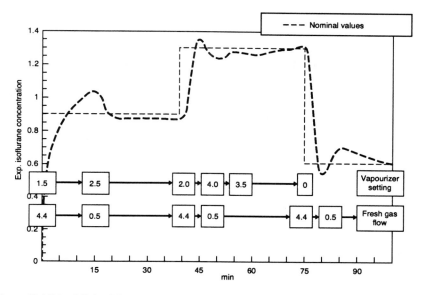

Figure 10.16(a)   Minimal flow anaesthesia: alteration of the expired isoflurane concentration to new desired nominal values by variation of fresh gas flow and vaporizer setting. Anaesthesia management with changing time constants (From Baum[15])

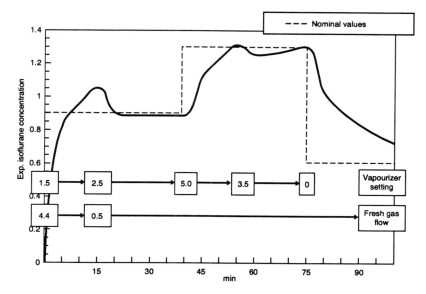

Figure 10.16(b)   Minimal flow anaesthesia: alteration of the expired isoflurane concentration to new desired nominal values only by variation of the vaporizer setting. Anaesthesia management maintaining long time constant (From Baum[15])

volume first has to be fed into the breathing system and the lungs by compressing the manual bag and keeping it squeezed before the ventilator is switched on.

Due to the long time constant and depending on the duration of anaesthesia, the admixture of isoflurane to the fresh gas can be ceased about 15–30 min before the intervention is completed, so long as the low flow is maintained. Continuing with low fresh gas flow, the patient is then subjected to assisted manual ventilation until spontaneous breathing is restored. Approximately 5–10 min prior to extubation, the anaesthetic gases are washed out of the system completely with an oxygen flow of 4–6 l/min after the APL valve has been opened and nitrous oxide administration ceased. Immediate postoperative care of the patient takes place in the usual manner.

It has always to be considered, however, that dosage of volatile anaesthetics should not be focused upon a certain concentration, but on the required anaesthetic depth. It is for this reason that this very simple standardized dosage scheme should only be regarded as a guideline, which has to be adjusted to individual requirements. Should any problems arise in performance of minimal flow anaesthesia, particularly for colleagues starting to deal with low flow anaesthetic techniques, it is recommended that the anaesthetist switches to familiar high fresh gas flows in the interest of patient safety. If however, a lower concentration of the selected inhalational anaesthetic is sought as the nominal value over the entire course of anaesthesia, the standard adjustments at the vaporizer should be made correspondingly lower for both the initial high flow, and the following minimal flow phase (Figures 10.17 and 10.18).

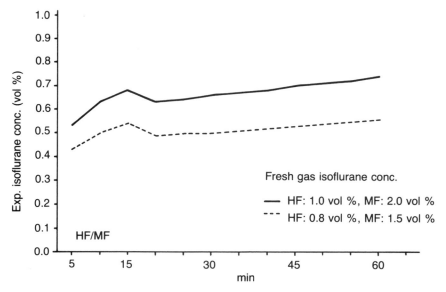

Figure 10.17   Expired isoflurane concentration during the course of minimal flow anaesthesia with lower standard settings of the vaporizer (Simulation using the 'Gas Uptake Simulation' computer program, assuming an adult patient with normal body weight; HF/MF, flow reduction from 4.4 to 0.5 l/min)

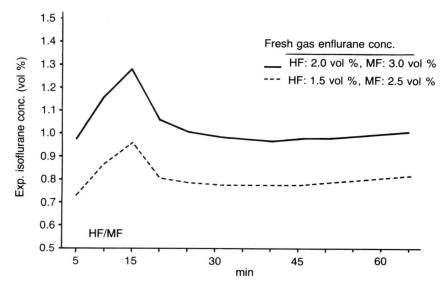

Figure 10.18   Expired enflurane concentration during the course of minimal flow anaesthesia with lower standard settings of the vaporizer (Simulation using the 'Gas Uptake Simulation' computer program, assuming an adult patient with normal body weight; HF/MF, flow reduction from 4.4 to 0.5 l/min)

Applying this easily manageable standardized dosage scheme facilitates considerably the performance of minimal flow anaesthesia. But it must be kept in mind that, by maintaining a given fresh gas composition during longer periods of time, one has to expect slow but continuous change of the gas composition within the breathing system[32]. However, based on experience gained during application of such standardized dosage schemes in routine clinical practice over a period of more than 10 years, the assessment is justified that this specific feature of minimal flow anaesthesia is neither disadvantageous nor clinically relevant, provided that the technique is followed appropriately.

10.5   The laryngeal mask airway

The laryngeal mask, which was introduced by Brain in 1983[33,34], is an entirely new concept of airway management. The device consists of a silicone mask formed to fit the anatomy of the hypopharynx and being attached to a silicone tube (Figure 10.19). The mask is available in six different sizes which makes it suitable for all age groups from the neonate to the large adult. The opening of the laryngeal mask is positioned over the laryngeal orifice. Once the sealing cuff is inflated, it provides an adequate seal to the airway. Computer tomographic investigations of the position revealed a perfect seal to the airways if the mask was inserted properly[35]. Handling of the device is simple and can be easily learned, but it must be admitted that it requires some training to become familiar with its use.

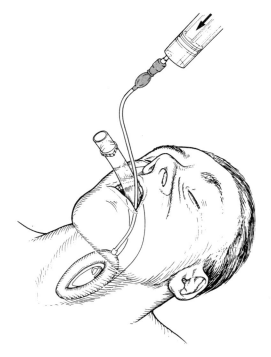

Figure 10.19   Laryngeal mask: correct position directly over the laryngeal orifice; the sealing cuff is inflated (from Brain[34], by permission)

The following are the advantages of this new airway, which is a link between the face mask and the endotracheal tube[36,37]:

- simple positioning without laryngoscopy, which means only minor circulatory reactions upon insertion
- accidental oesophageal or bronchial malpositioning is impossible
- insertion is less traumatic than with endotracheal intubation, improving the postoperative condition of the patient
- only minor irritation of the pharynx: after the initial phase, during which anaesthesia has to be sufficiently deep, the device is tolerated virtually to complete emergence
- diminished occurrence of laryngospasm compared with endotracheal intubation
- unhindered spontaneous breathing is guaranteed more reliably than via a conventional face mask
- provides safer protection from accidental aspiration than the face mask
- simplifies performance of anaesthesia, as the hands of the anaesthetist are kept free
- compared with the face mask, considerably facilitates monitoring with the aid of capnometry or measurement of the expired gas volume

● transition from spontaneous breathing to ventilation and vice versa is rendered very easy
● may be an alternative in cases of unexpected difficult endotracheal intubation.

It must be pointed out, on the other hand, that aspiration cannot reliably be precluded in the case of regurgitation, since endoscopy has revealed that in 6% of the cases the seal of the inflated cuff toward the oesophagus was insufficient[36]. However, it can be assumed that protection against aspiration is more reliable than in anaesthesia using a conventional face mask[36]. Controlled ventilation via the laryngeal mask is possible in most cases if the airway pressure does not exceed 17–20 cmH$_2$O.

In comparison with the conventional face mask, the better gas seal of the connection to the patient's airway is an essential advantage of the laryngeal mask. This lessens the contamination of the operating room atmosphere with anaesthetic gases, thus helping to satisfy the requirements of increasingly stringent regulations on occupational safety and health (see Section 6.3.1).

Furthermore, the use of the laryngeal mask facilitates the performance of low flow anaesthesia techniques in short-term surgical interventions on spontaneously breathing patients. During controlled ventilation, older type conventional anaesthetic machines work without an anaesthetic gas reservoir. This operating mode needs precise tuning of the fresh gas flow to that gas volume being lost by uptake and leaks (see Section 7.2.6) so as to prevent changes in ventilation. However, if these machines are used on spontaneously breathing patients, the manual bag, which is attached directly to the breathing system, assumes the function of a gas reservoir. In this way, performance of low flow anaesthesia is considerably simplified since adaptation of the fresh gas flow to the gas volume being lost is made much easier. Possible imbalances are compensated for by the changing degree of filling of the manual bag.

In the author's department, the laryngeal mask is exclusively used on patients with an empty stomach and for surgical interventions which, in principle, can be performed with spontaneous breathing. If, however, artificial ventilation can be carried out without problems, intermittent positive pressure ventilation (IPPV) or synchronized intermittent mandatory ventilation (SIMV) is used in order to prevent atelectasis. Initially, the sealing cuff is inflated with a volume according to the instructions for use.

In the author's department in 1994, nearly 20% of all cases undergoing inhalational anaesthesia were performed with the use of the laryngeal mask. The average duration of anaesthesia was about 55 min and minimal flow anaesthesia could be realized in about 85% of these cases, in spite of the fact that different modes of mechanical ventilation were applied on nearly 90% of the patients (Figure 10.20). The actual proportion of time during which a flow of 0.5 l/min was administered amounted to about 55%. But if minimal flow anaesthesia was performed with the laryngeal mask, the possibilities of flow reduction were used to their full potential since, on average, a high fresh gas flow was used for only about 18 min during the induction and recovery phase. Different methods of inhalational anaesthesia and the total proportion in time during which the flow was actually reduced to 0.5 l/min, respectively, are listed in Table 10.3.

The present author agrees with the clinical experience of other authors

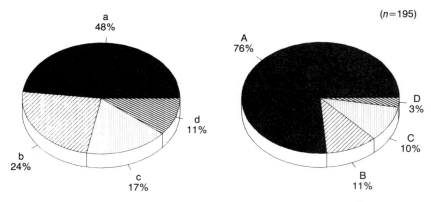

Figure 10.20 Minimal flow anaesthesia via the laryngeal mask. Left pie, ventilation mode (a, IPPV; b, SIMV; c, ventilation only with muscle relaxation; d, spontaneous breathing). Right pie, performance of minimal flow anaesthesia (A, without any problem; B, 1–2 × refilling of the gas reservoir; C, no attempt at flow reduction; D, flow reduction unsuccessful)

Table 10.3   Different techniques to perform inhalational anaesthesia (figures from the author's department, 1994)*

	A	B	C	D
Anaesthesia with face mask	13.0%	14.8 min	4.1%	3.1%
Anaesthesia with endotracheal intubation	67.3%	68.4 min	85.7%	61.2%
Anaesthesia with laryngeal mask	19.7%	55.7 min	87.5%	56.3%

* A, Incidence of respective technique, in relation to the total number of inhalation anaesthetics; B, average duration; C, proportion of cases performed with minimal flow anaesthesia, related to the respective technique; D, proportion of time during which the flow was reduced to 0.5 l/min, related to the total time performed with the respective technique.

that low flow anaesthetic techniques can be performed on most patients in whom the laryngeal mask airway is used[38,39]. A reduction in the use of face mask anaesthesia in favour of the laryngeal mask is recommended in order to reduce the workplace contamination by inhalational anaesthetics to an even greater extent.

The author's experiences can be summarized as follows. Barbiturates or propofol should be given in generous induction doses to achieve a deep initial anesthetic level together with an appropriate inhibition of reflexes. In most cases the laryngeal mask can be inserted without any problems. The correct position can easily be verified by checking whether manual ventilation can be carried out with only slight elastic resistance. Should insufflation be difficult and high pressures build up, the laryngeal mask has to be removed immediately and a new attempt made at insertion. In doing so it may be advisable to effect brief relaxation with a short acting muscle relaxant. For instance, during insertion the laryngeal mask may be or to use another technique. During insertion, the laryngeal mask is turned carefully by 90° like a Guedel airway. A moistened gauze bandage may be placed between the rows of teeth as a gag. Preferably, in the author's department, a special disinfectable device is used for bite protection (Figure 10.21a,b), fixing the tube

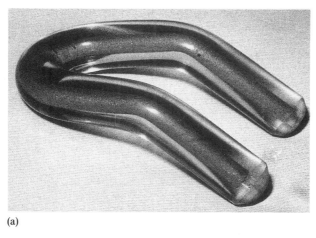

(a)

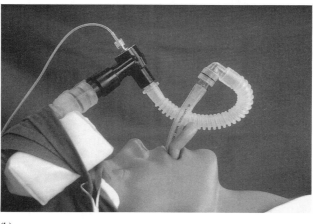

(b)

Figure 10.21 A simple gag which both protects against occlusion and ensures the correct position of the laryngeal mask airway (from Sachs and Baum[41]). Laryngeal mask airway and gag *in situ*. Smooth connection between the Y-piece and the tube connector via a short flexible silicon hose additionally ensures the correct position of the laryngeal mask[44] (from Baum and Sachs[40])

in the midline, thus providing an additional aid to proper positioning and sufficient sealing of the laryngeal mask[40,41]. Where elderly patients are concerned, it may happen in the individual case that the laryngeal mask dislocates spontaneously from its originally correct position into the oropharynx. This must be attributed to age-related atrophic alteration of the pharyngeal profile and reduced turgor of the tissues. The laryngeal mask is impressively well tolerated during emergence and may be kept in place until full awakening, which ensures optimum protection of unhindered spontaneous breathing.

The laryngeal mask is thus a valuable means of reduction of emission of inhalational anaesthetics. This new device facilitates low flow anaesthesia in short surgical interventions and also the performance of low flow techniques with conventional anaesthesia machines on spontaneously breathing patients.

10.6   Day-case surgery

If an attempt is made to adopt low flow techniques in very short surgical interventions, the following must be considered. An initial high fresh gas flow is needed to ensure adequate denitrogenation, achievement of the desired anaesthetic gas composition within the breathing system within the short time available and bridging of possible initial gas volume imbalances. For sufficient denitrogenation a flow of 4–6 l/min has to be used over a period of at least 6–8 min. The desired concentration of the volatile anaesthetic can only be achieved quickly by setting high fresh gas concentrations, so as to increase the alveolar–blood partial pressure difference, thus accelerating uptake of volatile anaesthetic. Nevertheless the problem of initially high nitrous oxide uptake with the resulting possibility of gas volume imbalance remains unresolved, if the flow is reduced to 0.5 l/min shortly after denitrogenation.

Stepwise reduction of the fresh gas flow may be an alternative method to adopt for low flow techniques even in very short anaesthetics. In the first 5 min the flow is set to 4.4 l/min (1.4 l/min O_2, 3.0 l/min N_2O), over the following period of 10 min to 1.0 l/min (0.4 l/min O_2, 0.6 l/min N_2O) and then to 0.5 l/min (0.25 l/min O_2, 0.25 l/min N_2O). Applying this flow control scheme, the vaporizer setting can be standardized to 3.0% for isoflurane (Figure 10.22) and to 4.0% for enflurane. But if this technique of stepwise flow

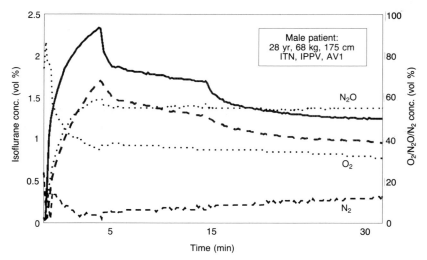

Figure 10.22   Course of anaesthetic gas composition during performance of short-term anaesthesia by stepwise control of the fresh gas flow (5 min: 4.4 l/min; 10 min.: 1.0 l/min; then 0.5 l/min); vaporizer setting maintained at 3% (male patient aged 28 yr, weight 68 kg, height 1.75 m). Computer-based on-line record, gas analyser: Capnomac (Datex, Helsinki, Finland)

reduction is judged honestly, no real advantage will be gained. During a 15-minute anaesthetic performed with stepwise flow reduction, only 24 litres of nitrous oxide but no volatile anaesthetic can be saved in comparison with minimal flow anaesthesia maintaining a high flow over an initial period of 15 min. Due to shortening of the wash-out phase, foreign gas as nitrogen will accumulate at a comparatively high level even after a short time. The technique is involved, as flow adjustment is required just at the time when the anaesthetist is occupied by setting of monitors, positioning of the patient and preparation for the surgical intervention. Accordingly, timely flow adjustments will often be omitted. And the better climatization of the anaesthetic gases, resulting from flow reduction, can only be gained after a certain time delay.

However, compared with high flow anaesthesia (4.4 l/min), if minimal flow anaesthesia is applied according to the aforementioned standardized scheme during an anaesthetic lasting only 60 min, 33.7% ($\simeq$ 11.80 US\$) of the overall costs of 58.08 DM ($\simeq$ 34.16 US\$) can be saved, in spite of the use of more expensive supplementary drugs like propofol, atracurium, alfentanyl and the use of the laryngeal mask. Even in a 30-min anaesthetic, 15% ($\simeq$ 4.10 US\$) of the total costs of 42.04 DM ($\simeq$ 24.72 US\$) can be saved by adequate use of available rebreathing equipment. Thus, if day-case surgery is performed under general anaesthesia with inhalational anaesthetics, low flow anaesthetic techniques should be applied whenever the surgical intervention lasts longer than 15 min.

10.7   Paediatric anaesthesia

As a rule, the techniques of low flow or minimal flow anaesthesia can be applied on all paediatric patients in whom use is made of a rebreathing system. Special paediatric circle absorber systems such as the Ulmer Kreissystem (Drägerwerk, Lübeck, Germany) are available for this purpose (Figure 10.23). Such systems feature appropriately small ventilation bellows, an absorber canister with reduced volume, a special scaled volumeter and a patient hose assembly with small diameter tubing characterized by very low compliance[42]. Paediatric anaesthesia with low fresh gas flow can be performed even more easily without any age restriction with the newer generation of anaesthetic machines such as the Cato and Cicero (Drägerwerk, Lübeck, Germany). The software controlling the ventilator operation permits setting of tidal volumes down to 20 ml. This enables the anaesthetist to use rebreathing systems even on newborns and very small infants.

The following advantages result from the use of rebreathing systems even in children with a body weight lower than 15 kg[43]:

- less pollution of the working place atmosphere with inhalational anaesthetics
- less emission of waste anaesthetic gases
- exact monitoring of ventilation parameters such as expired volume and airway pressure is rendered possible
- unrestricted possibility of carbon dioxide monitoring
- improved climatization of the anaesthetic gases

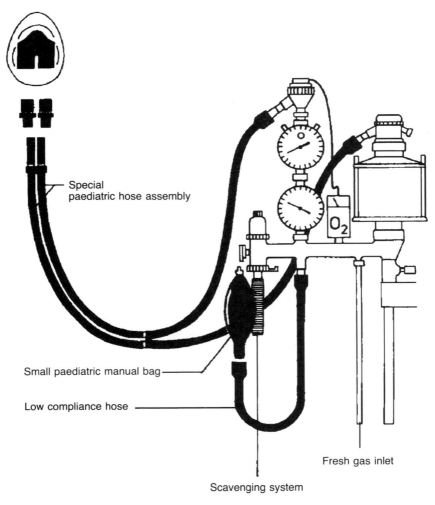

Special paediatric hose assembly

Small paediatric manual bag

Low compliance hose

Fresh gas inlet

Scavenging system

Figure 10.23   Ulmer-Kreissystem (Drägerwerk, Lübeck, Germany): Circle absorber system for use in paediatric anaesthesia (From Kretz and Striebel[43], by permission)

- less loss of heat and humidity
- possibility of controlled mechanical ventilation
- less liability to accidental carbon dioxide rebreathing
- considerable cost savings.

It must be considered, however, that in paediatric anaesthesia the total gas uptake is low compared with the fresh gas volume, even in the case of considerable flow reduction. Furthermore, the gas-containing space, consisting of the lungs, the breathing system and the ventilator volume, is comparatively small. Thus, the time constant is correspondingly short and changes in fresh gas composition take effect in the paediatric breathing system within a relatively short period of time.

As patient variability in response to volatile agent concentration is much more marked, standardized guidelines for the dosage of volatile anaesthetics in paediatric anaesthesia will not be proposed. Where enflurane is concerned, the fresh gas concentrations required for maintenance of adequate anaesthetic depth correspond almost exactly to the standards quoted for anaesthesia in adults. However, again it has to be pointed out that, with identical fresh gas concentration, the anaesthetic concentration gained in the breathing system will be considerably higher in paediatric than in adult anaesthesia.

Since the proportion in excess gas is comparatively high, which compensates for minor gas losses, low flow anaesthesia can also be performed with endotracheal tubes without a cuff if their size is selected appropriately. If anaesthetic machines with anaesthetic gas reservoirs are used, it is advisable to replace the special paediatric manual bag (0.5 litre), which is used during induction, by a manual bag with large volume (2.3 litres) prior to flow reduction. Thus, after flow reduction, a large gas volume will be available to compensate for possible gas volume imbalances. The manual bag should be detached from its mount and left resting freely to prevent unwanted gas loss via the excess gas discharge valve (see Section 10.4).

10.8   References

1. Virtue, R. W. Minimal flow nitrous oxide anesthesia. *Anesthesiology*, **40**, 196–198 (1974)
2. Bergmann, H. Das Narkosegerät in Gegenwart und Zukunft aus der Sicht des Klinkers. *Anaesthesist*, **35**, 587–594 (1986)
3. Baum, J. Contaminazione Batterica dei Sistemi Ventilatori. La Riduzione del Flusso Aumenta il Rischio? In *Anesthesia a Bassi Flussi e a Circuito Chiuso* (ed. F. Giunta), Piccin Nuova Libraria, Padova (1992), pp. 173–180
4. Baum, J., Enzenauer, J., Krausse, Th. and Sachs, G. Atemkalk – Nutzungsdauer, Verbrauch und Kosten in Abhängigkeit vom Frischgasfluß. *Anaesthesiol. Reanim.*, **18**, 108–113 (1993)
5. Bengtson, J. P., Brandberg, Å., Brinkhoff, B., Sonander, H. and Stenqvist, O. Low-flow anaesthesia does not increase the risk of microbial contamination through the circle absorber system. *Acta Anaesth. Scand.*, **33**, 89–92 (1989)
6. Deutsche Gesellschaft für Anästhesiologie und Intensivmedizin: Hygienische Maßnahmen als Bestandteil der Anwendungssicherheit medizinisch-technischer Geräte. *Anästh. Intensivmed.*, **24**, 79–82 (1984)
7. Mazze, R. I. Bacterial air filters. *Anesthesiology*, **54**, 359–360 (1981)
8. Luttropp, H. H. and Berntman, L. Bacterial filters protect anaesthetic equipment in a low-flow system. *Anaesthesia*, **48**, 520–523 (1993)
9. Kohler, P., Rimek, A., Albrecht, M., Frankenberger, H., Mertins, W. and Ackern, K.v. Sind Feuchtigkeitsfilter in der Inspirationsluft während der Narkose notwendig? *Anästhesiol. Intensivmed. Notfallmed. Schmerzther.*, **27**, 149–155 (1992)
10. Barton, F. J. and Nunn, F. Totally closed circuit nitrous oxide/oxygen anaesthesia. *Br. J. Anaesth.*, **47**, 350–357 (1975)
11. Parbrook, G. D. The levels of nitrous oxide analgesia. *Br. J. Anaesth.*, **39**, 974–982 (1967)
12. Parbrook, G. D. Therapeutic use of nitrous oxide. *Br. J. Anaesth.*, **40**, 365 (1968)
13. Don, H. Hypoxemia and hypercapnia during and after anesthesia. In *Complications in Anesthesiology* (eds F. K. Orkin and L. H. Cooperman), Lippincott, Philadelphia (1983), pp. 183–207
14. Westenskow, D. R. How much oxygen? *Int. J. Clin. Monitor. Comput.*, **2**, 187–189 (1986)

15. Baum, J. *Die Narkose mit niedrigem Frischgasfluß. Darstellung des Verfahrens in Frage und Antwort.* Bibliomed – Medizinische Verlagsanstalt, Melsungen (1993)
16. Arndt, J. O. Inhaltionsanästhetika und Stoffwechsel. O_2-Verbrauch wacher, schlafender oder narkotisierter Hunde unter Grundumsatzbedingungen. In *Die Inhalationsnarkose: Steuerung und Überwachung* (eds H. Schwilden and H. Stoeckel), INA-Schriftenreihe, Bd. 58, Thieme, Stuttgart (1987), pp. 43–52
17. Severinghaus, J. W. The rate of uptake of nitrous oxide in man. *J. Clin. Inv.*, **33**, 1183–1189 (1954)
18. Halsey, M. J. A reassessment of the molecular structure – functional relationships of the inhaled general anaesthetics. *Br. J. Anaesth.*, **56** (Suppl. !), 9S–25S (1984)
19. Terrell, R. C. Physical and chemical properties of anaesthetic agents. *Br. J. Anaesth.*, **56** (Suppl. 1), 3S–7S (1984)
20. Eger II, E. J. The pharmacology of isoflurane. *Br. J. Anaesth.*, **56** (Suppl. 1), 71S–99S (1984)
21. Baum, J. Minimal flow anaesthesia with isoflurane. In *Isoflurane. Anaesthesiologie und Intensivmedizin* (eds P. Lawin, H. van Aken, Ch. Puchstein), Bd. 182, Springer, Berlin (1986), pp. 325–331
22. Lowe, H. J. *Dose-Regulated Penthrane Anesthesia*, Abbott Laboratories, Chicago (1972)
23. Nemes, C., Niemer, M. and Noack, G. *Datenbuch Anästhesiologie*, Fischer, Stuttgart (1979)
24. Weiskopf, R. B. Inhalation anaesthetics: today and tomorrow. In *Update on Modern Inhalation Anaesthetics* (eds G. Torri, G. and G. Damia), Worldwide Medical Communications, New York (1989), pp. 23–28
25. Zbinden, A. M. *Inhalationsanästhetika: Aufnahme und Verteilung*, Wissenschaftliche Verlagsabteilung, Deutsche Abbott, Wiesbaden (1987)
26. Schwilden, H., Stoeckel, H., Lauven, P. M. and Schüttler, J. Pharmakokinetik und MAC – Praktische Implikationen für die Dosierung volatiler Anästhetika. In *Inhaltionsanaesthetika. Anaesthesiologie und Intensivmedizin* (eds K. Peter, B. R. Brown, E. Martin and O. Norlander), Bd. 184. Springer, Berlin (1986), pp. 18–26
27. Torri, G., Salvo, P., Righi, E., Calderini, E. and Bordoli, W. Pharmakokinetic profile of isoflurane in children. In *Isoflurane. Anaesthesiologie und Intensivmedizin* (eds P. Lawin, H. van Aken and Ch. Puchstein), Bd. 182. Springer, Berlin (1986), pp. 24–28
28. Robson, J. G., Gillies, ·D. M., Cullen, W. G. and Griffith, H. R. Fluothane (halothane) in closed circuit anesthesia. *Anesthesiology*, **20**, 251–260 (1959)
29. Bennets, N. B. Halothane and the liver – the problem revisited. In Proceedings of a Symposium at Bristol University Medical School, 11 April 1986, Sir Humphry Davy Department of Anaesthesia, Bristol Royal Infirmary (1986)
30. Brown Jr, B. R. and Gandolfi, A. J. Adverse effects of volatile anaesthetics. *Br. J. Anaesth.*, **59**, 14–23 (1987)
31. Hobbhahn, J., Hansen, E., Conzen, P. and Peter, K. Der Einfluß von Inhalationsanästhetika auf die Leber. *Anasth. Intensivmed.*, **32**, 215–220 and 250–256 (1991)
32. Gregorini, P. Effect of low fresh gas flow rates on inspired gas composition in a circle absorber system. *J. Clin. Anaesth.*, **4**, 439–443 (1992)
33. Brain, A. I. J. The laryngeal mask – a new concept in airway management. *Br. J. Anaesth.*, **55**, 801–805 (1983)
34. Brain, A. I. J. *The Intavent Laryngeal Mask*, Instruction Manual, Intavent (1990)
35. Calder, I., Ordman, A. J., Jackowski, A. and Crockard, H. A. The brain laryngeal mask airway. An alternative to emergency tracheal intubation. *Anaesthesia*, **45**, 137–139 (1990)
36. Leach, A. B. and Alexander, C. A. The laryngeal mask – an overview. *Eur, J. Anaesthesiol.* (Suppl. 4), 19–31 (1991)
37. Silk, J. M., Hill, H. M. and Calder, I. Difficult intubation and the laryngeal mask. *Eur. J. Anaesthesiol.* (Suppl. 4), 47–51 (1991)
38. Möllhoff, Th., Burgard, G. and Th. Prien, T. R. Low-Flow-Anästhesie während der Beatmung mit der laryngealen Maske. Anaesthesist, **42** (Suppl. 1), S141 (1993)
39. Stacey, M. R. W. and Shambrook, A. Laryngeal mask airway and low flow anaesthesia. *Anaesthesia*, **47**, 1108 (1992)

40. Baum, J. and Sachs, G. Comment on J. Brimacombe's statement 'The laryngeal mask airway – fixation, gags and stability'. *Anästhesiol. Intensivmed. Notfallmed. Schmerzther.*, **30**, 130 (1995)

41. Sachs, G. and Baum, J. Ein einfacher Beißschutz für die Kehlkopfmaske. *Anästhesiol. Intensivmed. Notfallmed. Schmerzther.*, **29**, 309–310 (1994)

42. Striebel, H. W. and Kretz, F.-J. Narkosesysteme. In *Basisinformationen Kinderanästhesia* (eds F.-J. Kretz and H. W. Striebel), Editiones Roche, Basel (1991), pp. 78–82

43. Kretz, F.-J. and Striebel, H. W. (eds) *Kinderanästhesie*, Editiones Roche, Basel (1991)

44. Brimacombe, J. The laryngeal mask airway – Fixation, gags and stability. *Anästhesiol. Intensivmed. Notfallmed. Schmerzther.*, **30**, 129 (1995)

Perspectives

11.1 Future technical developments

Currently available anaesthetic machines of the new generation, being equipped with adequate safety features and perfectly tight compact breathing systems, are designed for the utilization of rebreathing and the use of even the lowest fresh gas volumes. It may be assumed that in future electronic flow control and dosage systems will replace the conventional combination of fine needle valves, flowmeter tubes and plenum vaporizers, a concept which was realized for the first time in 1910 with Neu's nitrous oxide oxygen anaesthetic apparatus. This will facilitate not only the fresh gas flow independent dosage of volatile anaesthetics, but also the control of the dosage system itself by computer-controlled closed-loop feedback according to preselected nominal values for the anaesthetic gas composition. Such a technical concept has already been realized in the PhysioFlex anaesthetic machine (Physio, Haarlem, The Netherlands).

11.2 Environmental protection and occupational health and safety

The growing environmental awareness and increasingly stringent regulations on occupational safety and health make obligatory the judicious use of available anaesthetic equipment to reduce as far as possible the consumption of anaesthetic gases. The discussion on environmental pollution by inhalational anaesthetics will be even more accentuated in so far as, according to the London Protocol of 1990, the production of fully halogenated fluorochlorocarbons (CFCs) has to be ceased completely by the year 2000 at the latest. This means that the proportion of volatile anaesthetics in the total yearly production and consumption of CFCs will increase, which in turn raises the question of environmental compatibility of uncontrolled and unnecessary emission of anaesthetic gases. In view of these aspects, it can be expected that the future will bring even more stringent requirements for the most sparing use and perhaps even recycling of inhalational anaesthetics[1,2].

11.3   Future inhalational anaesthetics

A common tendency with respect to molecular structure can be observed in the development of new volatile anaesthetics[3]. The integration of halogen atoms will further ensure non-inflammability. The exclusively fluoro-substituted molecules feature great chemical stability, minimal metabolism and, according to present-day knowledge, a lower potential for ozone layer destruction. An ether analogue structure of the molecules results in a lower incidence of cardiac dysrhythmias. However, the anaesthetic potency of volatile anaesthetics of such molecular structure tends to be low; they are less soluble in blood and of higher volatility.

Due to the physicochemical properties of desflurane, for instance, the induction and recovery phase are very short[4]. In addition, the metabolism is significantly lower than that of isoflurane by a factor of 10.

At present, the cost of desflurane, adjusted for its lower potency, is significantly higher than that of isoflurane. The high volatility of this agent with a vapour pressure of 664 mmHg at 22°C requires special vaporizers. The fact that the anaesthetic potency of desflurane is only one-fifth that of isoflurane necessitates considerably higher concentrations in the anaesthetic gas. The amount of anaesthetic vapour discharged into the atmosphere, together with the excess gas, is about five times higher than during isoflurane anaesthesia, making the use of desflurane in high flow anaesthesia an extremely uneconomical proposition[5].

Due to the low solubility of desflurane the amount of this agent, taken up by the patient after initial wash-in, is comparatively low, facilitating the control of this agent during low flow anaesthesia. If a fresh flow of 1 l/min is used, the inspired desflurane concentration nearly equals the concentration in the fresh gas[12]: 'What you set is what you get'. The author's early and limited clinical experiences using desflurane in minimal flow anaesthesia can be summarized as follows (Figures 11.1 and 11.2):

- During the initial high flow phase, as soon as 10 minutes after induction the F_I/F_D ratio, the quotient formed by the division of the inspired concentration (F_I) by the delivered concentration (F_D), gains a value between 0.95–0.88 and the F_E/F_D (F_E: expired concentration) ratio between 0.84–0.78. In the following 5 minutes the additive increments of the quotients, i.e. F_I/D_D to 0.96–0.9 and F_E/F_D to 0.86–0.81, are negligible. With the use of desflurane the initial high flow phase can be kept as short as possible, and is determined mainly by the initial high nitrous oxide and the time needed for sufficient wash-out of nitrogen.
- There is only a slight decrease of the in- and expired desflurane concentration after flow reduction from 4.4 to 0.5 l/min if the fresh gas concentration is kept constant. In 20 minutes, following flow reduction, the F_I/F_D decreases to 0.84–0.79 and the F_E/F_D to 0.77–0.73. This decrease of the in- and expired concentrations can be compensated for if the delivered desflurane concentration is increased by 1% at lower, or 2% at higher inspired nominal desflurane concentrations respectively.
- If the flow is kept constant at 0.5 l/min but the vaporizer setting increased by only 1%, there is a slow but continuous increase of the in- and expired concentration in the following 50 minutes. However, assuming only small

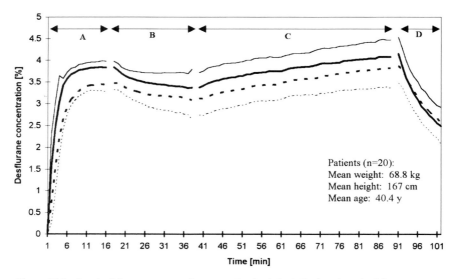

Figure 11.1 Inspired (——: mean and mean + standard deviation) and expired (------: mean and mean – standard deviation) desflurane concentration during minimal flow anaesthesia. A, 4.41 l/min, 4% desflurane; B, 0.5 l/min, 4% desflurane; C, 0.5 l/min, 5% desflurane; D, 0.5 l/min, 0% desflurane. (On-line registration, Cicero EM (Drägerwerk, Lübeck, Germany))

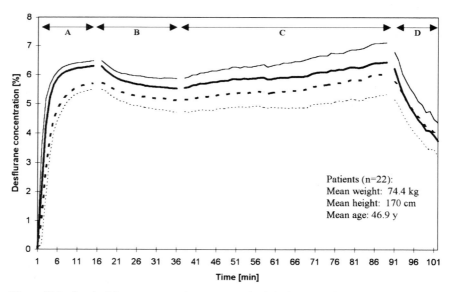

Figure 11.2 Inspired (——: mean and mean + standard deviation) and expired (------: mean and mean – standard deviation) desflurane concentration during minimal flow anaesthesia. A, 4.41 l/min, 7% desflurane; B, 0.5 l/min, 7% desflurane; C, 0.5 l/min, 8% desflurane; D, 0.5 l/min, 0% desflurane. (On-line registration, Cicero EM (Drägerwerk, Lübeck, Germany))

changes of the fresh gas desflurane concentration, the specifically long time constant of minimal flow anaesthesia still has to be kept in mind. However, the long time constant can be overcome, if desflurane is used, as the output of the vaporizer can be increased to 18%. In this way, the amount of desflurane delivered into the breathing system can readily be increased, compared with the small amount of desflurane taken up by the patient. Thus, even in minimal flow anaesthesia, it will be possible to increase the desflurane concentration quickly although keeping the flow constant in this low range.

• If the vaporizer is closed, in- and expired desflurane concentrations drop by 1.5–2.5% in the following 10 minutes. However, coasting to lower concentrations during the emergence phase is possible as with the other higher soluble volatiles. The wash-out of desflurane will be completed rapidly when the flow is increased to 4–6 l/min.

Its low solubility makes desflurane a nearly ideal volatile anaesthetic for low and minimal flow anaesthesia. The agent concentration delivered to the patient can be judged sufficiently precisely by the concentration set at the vaporizer. The long time constant of the low flow breathing system can be overcome by the rapid wash-in and wash-out of this agent and the high output of the vaporizer. Due to its low anaesthetic potency and low solubility, large amounts of desflurane vapour have only to be delivered into the breathing system so to establish the required high alveolar partial pressure, not to meet a correspondingly high uptake. Thus, as already emphasized, the use of this agent only can be justified if it is applied with one of the low flow anaesthetic techniques[13].

These considerations are valid even more for the rare gas xenon which was used as an anaesthetic for the first time by Cullen and Gross[6]. The properties of this inert gas are evaluated as being excellent. Its extremely low solubility in blood ensures short induction and recovery times. Given as a mixture with 30% O_2, xenon features an excellent analgesic potency and its use has no side-effects on haemodynamics and lung compliance[6–9]. All these advantages would make xenon a virtually ideal anaesthetic. It presents, however, only a small fraction of atmospheric air (0.8×10^{-5}% by vol) and for use as an anaesthetic it is extremely expensive at a price of about 7–15 US$ per litre[10].

From the economical and logistical viewpoint, the use of xenon as an inhalational anaesthetic would be justifiable only with the proviso that it is administered via a closed or recycling rebreathing system[10].

11.4   Improvements in patient care

Low flow anaesthesia results in a distinct improvement of the anaesthetic gas climate. This protects the function and the morphological integrity of the respiratory epithelium and reduces humidity and heat losses. The effect can be achieved simply by judicious use of available anaesthesia machines equipped with a rebreathing system. The use of supplementary heat and moisture exchangers confers no additional benefit and, being disposable items, they merely increase the problem of waste and expense.

Continuous measurement of oxygen uptake in quantitative closed system anaesthesia may pave the way for new dimensions in patient monitoring, permitting the early detection of subtle changes in hamodynamics and metabolism. Simultaneous measurement of the arterial and mixed venous oxygen contents may facilitate continuous monitoring of the cardiac output in accordance with the Fick principle.

11.5   Conclusions

All the arguments put forward speak in favour of a judicious use of rebreathing systems by consistent reduction of the fresh gas flow. Technically advanced anaesthetic machines featuring appropriate safety facilities including the required monitoring are already available. Further development will facilitate quantitative closed system anaesthesia. Anaesthetists should not close their eyes to this development, but rather should study the theoretical background and practical management of low flow anaesthetic techniques to the benefit of their patients and the environment[11].

11.6   References

1. Marx, Th., Gross-Alltag, F., Ermisch, J., Hähnel, J., Weber, L. and Friesdorf, W. Experimentelle Untersuchungen zur Rückgewinnung von Narkosegasen. *Anaesthesist*, **41**, 99–102 (1992)
2. Waterson, C. K. Recovery of waste anesthetic gases. In *Future Anesthesia Delivery Systems. Contemporary Anesthesia Practice* (eds B. R. Calkins and R. J. Saunders), F. A. Davies, Philadelphia (1984), pp. 109–124
3. Weiskopf, R. B. Inhalation anaesthetics today and tomorrow. In *Update on Modern Inhalation Anaesthetics* (eds G. Torri and G. Damia), Worldwide Medical Communications, New York (1980), pp. 23–28
4. Saidman, L. J. The role of desflurane in the practice of anesthesia. *Anesthesiology*, **74**, 399–401 (1991)
5. Weiskopf, R. B. and Eger II, E. I. Comparing the costs of inhaled anesthetics. *Anesthesiology*, **79**, 1413–1418 (1993)
6. Cullen, S. C. and Gross, E. G. The Anesthetic properties of xenon in animals and human beings, with observations on krypton. *Science*, **113**, 580–582 (1951)
7. Boomsma, F., Rupreht, J., Man In't Veld, A. J., De Jong, F. H., Dzoljic, M. and Lachmann, B. Haemodynamic and neurohumoral effects of xenon anaesthesia. *Anaesthesia*, **45**, 273–278 (1990)
8. Lachmann, B., Armbruster, S., Schairer, W. *et al.* Safety and efficacy of xenon in routine use as an inhalational anaesthetic. *Lancet*, **335**, 1413–1415 (1990)
9. Pittinger, C. B. The first Xenon anesthesia for surgery conducted with a closed absorption system. *Circular*, **3**, 19–20 (1986)
10. Luttropp, H. H., Rydgren, G., Thomasson, R. and Werner, O. A minimal-flow system for xenon anesthesia. *Anesthesiology*, **75**, 896–902 (1991)
11. Baum, J. Sind 'Niedriger Fluß' und 'Geschlossenes System' die Techniken der Zukunft? In *Inhalationsanästhesie – eine Standortbestimmung* (eds H. Laubenthal, C. Puchstein and C. Sirtl), (1991), pp. 30–43, Wissenschaftliche Verlagsabteilung Abbott, Wiesbaden
12. Hargasser, S., Hipp, R., Breinbauer, B., Mielke, L., Entholzer, E. and Rust, M. A lower solubility recommends the use of desflurane more than isoflurane, halothane, and enflurane under low-flow conditions. *J. Clin. Anaesth.*, **7**, 49–53 (1995)
13. Baum, J. A. and Aitkenhead, A. R. Low-flow anaesthesia. *Anaesthesia*, **50** (Suppl.), 37–44 (1995)

Index